PRAISE FOR *AGELESS VEGAN*

"*Ageless Vegan* is beautifully written and deliciously inspiring. With warmth and grace, *Ageless Vegan* makes the exceptional accessible with a light touch and deep truth. Ranging from familiar and comfortable to adventurous and sophisticated, the 100 delectable recipes are absolutely to live for! Let the motivating and transformational powers of *Ageless Vegan* be your guide to a life that glows."
—DAWN MONCRIEF, FOUNDING DIRECTOR OF A WELL-FED WORLD

"I love and recommend *Ageless Vegan*. This wonderful book empowers and inspires readers to live mindfully and healthfully and to make our world a kinder place. The authors, mother and daughter Mary and Tracye McQuirter, have been vegan for decades and they are glowing examples for the rest of us who aspire to lead healthy, happy and conscientious lives."
—GENE BAUR, AUTHOR OF *LIVING THE FARM SANCTUARY LIFE*, FOUNDER OF FARM SANCTUARY

"Filled with tasty recipes and an easy-to-follow meal plan, this book also tells a story of two truly amazing women who are dedicated to living their truest expression of themselves. Working toward making this world a better place also extends to what we put into our bodies, and Tracye makes this point through practical advice, in a way that will motivate you to see that healthy eating is empowering in so many ways."
—LIZ ROSS, CO-FOUNDER OF VEGAN ADVOCACY INITIATIVE

"Tracye McQuirter is committed to a more socially just world, and she sees food, nutrition and health as a key ingredient of such a world. Importantly, Tracye and her wonderful mom speak in this book with an informed but also compassionate voice. I believe this combination of expertise and compassion is key to building a better world, especially when helping people through personal dietary and lifestyle change. I highly recommend this book as a resource to anyone wanting to explore the life-changing benefits of plant-based nutrition."
—NELSON CAMPBELL, DIRECTOR AND WRITER, *PLANTPURE NATION*, FOUNDER OF PLANTPURE, INC. AND PLANTPURE COMMUNITIES, INC.

"No matter your age, gender, or background, *Ageless Vegan* is sure to inspire you to live your best life. Tracye and Mary prove that you can go vegan and maintain a vegan lifestyle at any age. They show how effortless, fulfilling, and delicious eating plants can be. This book isn't just for folks who are new to plant-based living; even longtime vegans will be inspired and delighted by the McQuirters' stories and fantastic recipes!"
—JENNÉ CLAIBORNE, AUTHOR OF *SWEET POTATO SOUL*

"Tracye and Mary McQuirter are an amazing and dynamic vegan daughter and mother I've known for almost 20 years. They both show the incredible benefits of being vegan, a the many ways being vegan helps people age healthfully, functionally, and beautifully.'
—MILTON MILLS, MD, CRITICAL CARE PHYSICIAN AND FEATURED MEDICAL AND NUTRITION EXPERT IN *WHAT THE HEALTH*

AGELESS VEGAN

AGELESS VEGAN

The SECRET to
LIVING A LONG
and HEALTHY
PLANT~BASED LIFE

TRACYE McQUIRTER, MPH
with MARY McQUIRTER

Da Capo

LIFE
LONG

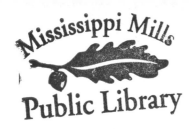

Food photography and styling by Kate Lewis

Author photography by a little bit of whimsy photography.

Da Capo Press
Hachette Book Group
1290 Avenue of the Americas, New York, NY 10104
dacapopress.com
@DaCapoPress

Printed in the United States of America

First Edition: June 2018

Published by Da Capo Press, an imprint of Perseus Books, LLC, a subsidiary of Hachette Book Group, Inc.

The Hachette Speakers Bureau provides a wide range of authors for speaking events. To find out more, go to www.hachettespeakersbureau.com or call (866) 376-6591.

The publisher is not responsible for websites (or their content) that are not owned by the publisher.

Print book interior design by Tara Long.

Library of Congress Cataloging-in-Publication Data
Names: McQuirter, Tracye Lynn, author. | McQuirter, Mary, author.
Title: Ageless vegan: the secret to living a long and healthy plant-based life / by Tracye McQuirter, MPH, with Mary McQuirter.
Description: First edition. | New York, NY: Hachette Book Group, 2018. |
Includes bibliographical references and index.
Identifiers: LCCN 2017058055| ISBN 9780738220208 (pbk.) | ISBN 9780738220215 (e-book)
Subjects: LCSH: Vegan cooking. | LCGFT: Cookbooks.
Classification: LCC TX837 .M47757 2018 | DDC 641.5/636—dc23
LC record available at https://lccn.loc.gov/2017058055

ISBNs: 978-0-7382-2020-8 (trade paperback); 978-0-7382-2021-5 (e-book)

LSC-C

10 9 8 7 6 5 4 3 2 1

Thank you, Dick Gregory.
Your legacy lives on.

TABLE of CONTENTS

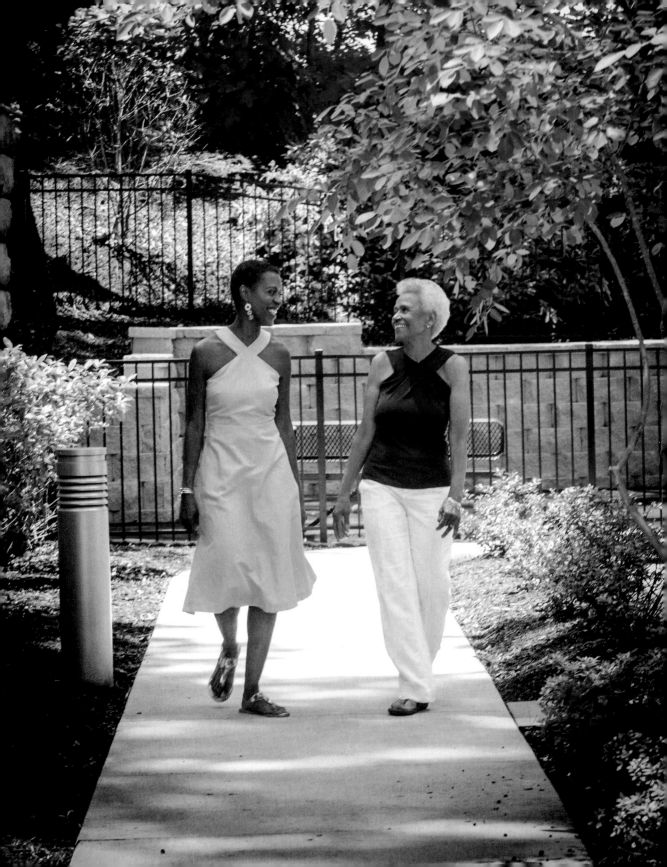

part one

VIBRANTLY VEGAN

Thirty Years and Counting

This book is a celebration. It's a toast to thirty years of being healthy, vibrant vegans and loving it. And it's an affirmation that a healthy vegan lifestyle can help keep you ageless. And by ageless, we simply mean living free from the diet-related diseases and decline most commonly associated with growing older.

So on this, our thirtieth vegan anniversary, what better way to mark the occasion than by sharing how we've done it, the tips we've learned along the way, and 100 of our favorite healthy and delicious vegan recipes that have kept us looking and feeling ageless for all these years?

We're grateful to be glowing examples of the long-term benefits of eating a whole food, plant-based diet. We went vegan in 1988, when I was twenty and my mother, Mary, was fifty. We're now fifty and eighty, but most people think we look fifteen to twenty years younger.

We're living proof that it's normal to be healthy and disease-free not only while we're younger, but as we get older, too. And the key is a healthy lifestyle. Eating more whole plant-based foods, along with exercising at least 30 minutes day, being smoke-free, and maintaining a healthy weight can reduce the risk of developing chronic diseases by nearly 80 percent, according to research published in the *Archives of Internal Medicine* in 2009. And of these lifestyle factors, eating healthy foods is the most important in preventing chronic diseases and premature disability and death, according to a landmark Global Burden of Diseases study published in the *Journal of the American Medical Association* in 2013.

So in this book, we show you how to go vegan for optimal health and longevity. We share our Fab Five Food Rules that serve as the foundation for what we eat every day, as well as particular superfoods that can ward off the diseases associated with aging. We also provide a guide we call "Fourteen Steps to a Healthier You," with practical, easy-to-follow advice on how to transition to vegan foods and jumpstart your healthy eating habits—and how to up your healthy eating game if you're already a vegan. To get you started cooking healthier right away, we also walk you through must-have kitchen tools and pantry staples to help you set up your vegan kitchen with ease and confidence.

Most importantly, we share 100 fresh, simple, and flavorful vegan recipes that can help *you* look and feel ageless, too. They're our favorite go-to dishes for everyday meals and special occasion treats, including Maple French Toast with Strawberries, Thai Coconut Curry Soup, Vegetable Pot Pie, Citrusy Dandelion Greens Salad, and Perfect Pecan Pie. All of our recipes use delicious and nutritious whole food ingredients—no highly processed foods, refined grains, or white sugar—because that's our secret to staying healthy and vibrant for the past thirty years.

With *Ageless Vegan*, our goal is to give you information, inspiration, and affirmation to live a long and healthy plant-based life you love.

But before we give you the *how*, we want to share with you our stories.

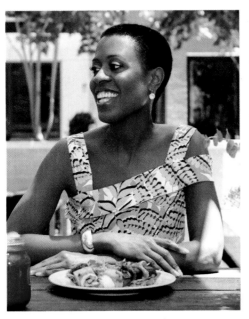

TRACYE'S JOURNEY

I absolutely love my vegan lifestyle. It's a liberating, joyful, and delicious way of living in the world. I get to eat good food that's good *for* me–and that's also good for other people, animals, and the planet. What could be better?

But the funny thing is I never thought I'd be a vegan. Growing up, I hated vegetables! I was always the last one left at the kitchen table pushing the green stuff around on my plate until my mother came back in the kitchen and put her foot down. Then I'd gulp them down and we'd go through the same thing again the next night.

My mother was pretty health conscious (as she talks about later in this chapter), so for my two sisters and me, that meant that although we ate meat and dairy, there was not a lot of processed food or junk food in the house. We ate relatively healthfully during the week and we got to splurge on the weekends. One of our favorite Saturday night dinners was smoked sausage, along with Kraft macaroni and cheese, Jiffy cornbread, butter pecan ice cream, and ginger ale. (Check out our healthier, vegan versions of these recipes in part 2 for Mac and Cheese, Southern-Style Cornbread, Maple Pecan Ice Cream, and Sparkling Basil Limonade.) We did have cousins and friends who had all the sodas, candy, and chips we could ever want, so we made up for it when we visited them. And at school there was an all-you-can eat cafeteria, so I could eat as many French fries and desserts as I wanted.

So it was my mother who first instilled in me the idea of healthy eating. But despite her best efforts, I liked the unhealthier food more. When I went off to Amherst College at seventeen, I gained twenty-five pounds my first year because I was away from home for the first time and could eat anything unhealthy I wanted, whenever I wanted.

HOW I BECAME A VEGAN

During my sophomore year at college, our Black Student Union brought civil rights movement icon and legendary comedian Dick Gregory to campus to talk about the state of black America. But instead, he decided to talk about the plate of black America, and how unhealthfully most folks eat. This was in 1986 and we didn't know that Gregory had become a vegetarian activist because of his practice of nonviolence during the Civil Rights Movement, which he extended to humans and animals alike.

During his two-hour talk, Gregory graphically traced the path of a hamburger from a cow on a factory farm, through the slaughterhouse process, to a fast-food restaurant, to a clogged artery, to a heart attack. And it rocked my world.

I was already going through a paradigm shift at the time. I was taking political science and African American studies classes, and I was learning about imperialism, racism, sexism, and more for the first time or in new ways, and it was changing my awareness and sense of self. And it was with this new consciousness that I listened to Dick Gregory's lecture. I was ready and open to questioning the way society dictated I should eat, as well.

After Gregory's lecture, I immediately gave up meat—which only lasted about a week. But I couldn't get what he said off my mind. I called my mother and one of my sisters, Marya, who was a senior at nearby Tufts University, and told them I thought I should become a vegetarian.

When I went home for the summer a few months later, I read every book I could find about vegetarianism in the local libraries, and my mother and sister read them with me. And by the end of the summer, we all decided to go vegetarian.

Well, as it turns out, it wasn't that easy. When school started again, I studied abroad for the first semester in Nairobi, Kenya, with twenty-nine other college students. It was one of the most incredible experiences of my life. But I was showing up as a new vegetarian and they weren't prepared to accommodate me so I still had to eat meat. While there, two life-altering incidents happened that made me know I would become a vegetarian again when I returned home.

The first happened when we lived and traveled for two weeks with Samburus, who are semi-nomadic pastoralists living in the northern plains of Kenya. One night, we stayed on a mountain cave and brought two live goats with us that we were going to eat. The day before, while staying with a Samburu family, I saw a goat being born, up close and personal. I was a nineteen-year-old city girl who'd never had a pet, and this was the first time I'd ever seen an animal give birth. It was amazing.

Well, the next day on the mountain cave, I watched the Samburu men slit the throat of one of the goats that we brought with us. They drank the blood that poured from its neck and invited us, as their guests, to do the same. Many

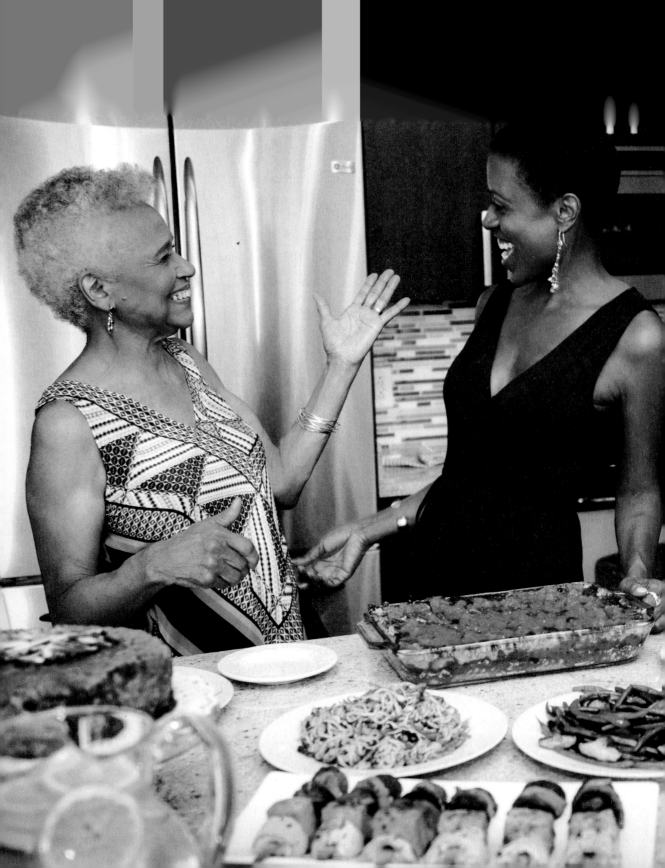

of the students did, and I was about to, as well, but I changed my mind at the last minute. The idea of actually drinking blood was too much.

The Samburu men then proceeded to skin and chop the goat to make stew. I don't remember actually watching them do that part, but I do remember looking over at the other goat that was tethered to a tree nearby and feeling sorry for it. I decided I wasn't going to eat the stew. But as we were passing the bowls to each other, it looked and smelled delicious, and I decided to eat it. But for the first time, I felt guilty about eating another animal. I wondered if the other goat knew what had happened to its companion.

A few days later, we went on safari at nearby Masai Mara. While there, we ate at a restaurant called The Carnivore, and the waiters brought out a large gazelle-looking animal that had been roasted over a pit. As they began to carve it in front of us from head to hoof, I became repulsed by it. And I knew in that moment that I never wanted to eat another animal again.

The next semester I went to Howard University in my hometown of Washington, DC. My mother and I spent much of that semester experimenting with vegetarian recipes we collected from newspapers, magazines, and vegetarian cookbooks. While I was at Howard, I was thrilled to discover that there was a large black vegan and vegetarian community just a few blocks from campus that had opened the first all-vegan cafes and health food stores in the nation's capital in the early 1980s.

This diverse community included longtime activists from the civil rights and black liberation movements, natural health entrepreneurs, raw foodists, Black Hebrew Israelites, the Ausar Auset Society, Muslims, college students, artists, and many more. And their influence was felt throughout the city at cultural festivals, Kwanzaa celebrations, and social justice rallies, where vegan food was the main fare.

I immersed myself in this community for nearly a year, soaking up their knowledge. I went to lectures, took cooking classes and learned where to shop, how to make it affordable, the politics of food, and much more. By the time I returned to Amherst for my senior year in the fall of 1987, I was a confident vegetarian. I wasn't ready to let go of cheese, so I wasn't vegan yet. Unfortunately, the dining hall at Amherst that served vegetarian options included eggs and cow's milk as ingredients, which I no longer ate, so that was not an option for me.

I had already sent a letter to the dean of students during the summer asking to be taken off of the meal plan so I could use that money to buy my own vegetarian food. But the dean had rejected my request, saying that students were required to be on the meal plan to ensure they were eating adequately and to foster socialization with other students. I decided to visit the dean when I got to campus to press my case further.

As I sat across from his desk, we went back and forth about the meal plan, with neither of us budging on our positions. Finally, I said that if I had to stay on the meal plan, I wanted the cafeteria to make separate vegetarian meals just for me, based on a menu that I provide, using organic ingredients, and separate pots and utensils. And that I wanted to watch them do it so I'd know they were doing it right. I figured he'd reject that idea completely and just take me off the meal plan. But instead, he called my bluff and agreed. He told me to bring him a menu and we'd start the following week.

So the next week, I showed up in the sweltering basement kitchen of the main cafeteria. I sat and watched as an unhappy cook made a tofu and vegetable stir-fry over brown rice on a cooktop in front of me. I tried to make small talk, but he barely spoke to me. When the rice finished cooking, about 45 minutes later, he handed me my plate of food, and I carried it upstairs to eat with my friends. By that time, they had almost finished eating.

Ultimately, being vegan makes me feel free. I know many people think being vegan means feeling restricted and deprived. But in reality, the opposite is true.

For dinner that day, I went back down to the hot kitchen and waited again while the cook made my food. I realized the whole thing was ridiculous and there was no way I could do that for the rest of the year. So I quietly took myself off the meal plan. I used some of the money I had saved from my summer job and money I was making from work-study to buy my own food.

Once a week, I caught the bus to the natural food store in town to buy groceries. Then I cooked my meals in the kitchen of the Charles Drew House where I lived, and carried my plate of food over to the cafeteria to eat with my friends. I did this twice a day for lunch and dinner.

But it gets cold up in Massachusetts, and many days I knew my hot plate of food would get cold by the time I walked to the cafeteria. So I stayed in Drew House and sat and ate in front of the TV. I felt alone without my community of support back home and I didn't know any other vegetarians or vegans on campus. But I remained committed to my vegetarianism because I knew I was doing it for my health and it was now a part of my lifestyle.

During my senior year, I decided to finally let go of cheese. That decision was purely mind over matter. I had to decide that the momentary pleasure of a piece of cheese in my mouth was not worth the health risks. I knew that cheese was the biggest source of artery-clogging saturated fat in the American diet. And I knew about the cruelty involved in using cows to make cheese. And yet cheese still looked and smelled good to me. So I had to come to terms with the fact that I might always love cheese, and that I might never be repulsed by it, like I was with meat. Once I accepted that fact, I gradually stopped obsessing about it, and the desire to eat it finally left me. There was no big, flashy moment when that happened. I just realized one day that I didn't want to eat cheese anymore. And so I became a full-fledged vegan. That was in 1988, soon after I graduated from college.

My mother and sister were also transitioning from vegetarian to vegan and we were all supporting each other. Being in this together as a family, and in a supportive larger community in DC, was the foundation that helped keep us going strong.

CHANGES I EXPERIENCED AFTER GOING VEGAN

After I became a vegan, the twenty-five pounds I gained during my first year at Amherst (the year before Dick Gregory's lecture) came off naturally. My menses also became lighter and shorter, and I seldom had cramps.

Growing up, I always had issues with oily skin and pimples, but even after becoming a vegan, my skin didn't clear up until I went on my first supervised cleanse, which included eating and drinking only raw vegan foods, particularly dark-green leafy vegetables. Within about two weeks, my skin cleared up and developed a healthy glow from the inside out. I've been able to maintain that glow, and good health in general, all these years because I still eat whole foods (including dark-green leafy vegetables three times a day) and cook from scratch.

I've now been a healthy vegan for all of my adult life. And now, at age fifty, I'm grateful that I haven't experienced any major health challenges. No high blood pressure, high cholesterol, diabetes, cancer, or any other chronic disease issues. Although being a vegan is not a get-out-of-disease-free card, since genetic and environmental factors are also involved, eating healthy plant-based foods gives me the best chance of living a long, healthy, and disease-free life.

In addition to the physical health benefits I experienced after going vegan, I also extended my veganism to express more compassion for and nonviolence toward animals. I served as a public policy liaison for the Physicians Committee for Responsible Medicine in 1999. As part of my role there, I watched undercover footage of factory farming; the wool and leather industries; circuses and zoos; and the testing of cosmetics, skincare, and household products on animals. I saw that the cruelty involved in using animals for fashion, furnishings, entertainment, and product testing was just as wrong as the cruelty involved in eating them. As a result, for the past twenty years, in addition to not eating animals, I also have not worn or used animal products in clothing or furnishings, and I have not used products tested on animals, to the best of my ability.

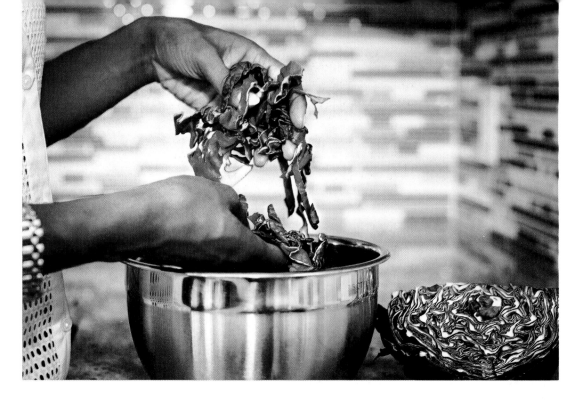

Being vegan has also strengthened my activism. Thanks to my mother's example, our family has long been involved in volunteer work in small and large ways to help improve the lives of people in our communities, and of people of color and poor people, in general. And in our early vegan years in the early 1990s, when we participated in antiwar marches and local social justice activities with our omnivore friends, many of them would go to fast-food restaurants to eat afterwards. Marya and I would have conversations with them about the intertwined oppressions of social injustice, poor health, and the food industry (you can read more about that in my book *By Any Greens Necessary*), but many of our friends did not make the connection. That was tough. I believed then and still do now that how we nourish ourselves is inextricably linked to every aspect of how we live our lives, including being activists for justice and equality.

And on the subject of activism, growing up I thought that I would be a writer, an investigative journalist, or a lawyer for the NAACP Legal Defense Fund or the ACLU. As it turned out, becoming a vegan led me to pursue activism as a public health nutritionist helping people take back control of their health and live longer, healthier, happier lives. Marya and I also started one of the earliest vegan websites, back in 1997, and I went on to direct the country's first federally funded and community-based vegan nutrition program in 2004, among some other milestones.

And finally, and most importantly, being vegan has also led me to explore other healing and self-care practices. As a result, I've developed a daily practice I call my Sacred Seven: meditating, exercising, journaling, expressing gratitude, eating well, having fun, and helping others. I've also gained greater clarity of purpose in my life. In fact, the longer I've been vegan, the more I understand that being vegan is a path, a practice—not a destination. It has served as an affirming foundation and template for me to live my life to the fullest.

WHY I LOVE BEING A VEGAN

Ultimately, being vegan makes me feel free. I know many people think being vegan means feeling restricted and deprived. But in reality, the opposite is true. Because of what I eat, I'm living a life that's healthiest for me and kindest to people, animals, and the planet. There's incredible freedom and fulfillment in that.

I also love the fact that being vegan and choosing the field of veganism as a profession have allowed me to combine my passions for writing, social justice, good food, travel, style, speaking, culture, and community building. Being a vegan is one of the beautiful and powerful lenses through which I see and live in the world and I feel incredibly grateful for that.

And, along with all of this, one of the biggest highlights of being a vegan has been the fact that my mother and sister went vegan with me. With my mother, in particular, we've come full circle. She planted the earliest seeds by starting us off on a healthier diet as children (although I didn't appreciate it at the time!). And for her to go vegan with me years later—and become a healthy, vibrant, vegan role model at eighty—has been amazing!

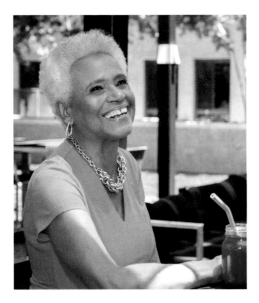

MARY'S STORY

My mother, Mary McQuirter, is a true inspiration. She went vegan with me thirty years ago, when she was fifty years old. And today, she's still healthy, fit, and active at eighty. She has no chronic diseases and takes no medications. In fact, her doctors tell her she has the health markers of someone thirty years younger. Here, my mother tells the story of how she went vegan and how it changed her life.

MY EARLY YEARS

I grew up on a farm in Camden, South Carolina, in the 1930s and 40s. We grew all our own fruits and vegetables, like kale, collards, sweet potatoes, green beans, watermelon, strawberries, and many more. And my Aunt Mary had a farm next to ours with an orchard full of peaches, plums, and all types of apples. We also picked wild blackberries and grapes in the woods that my mother preserved to make jam. We raised chickens, cows, and pigs, but we didn't eat meat every day, like we did with fruits and vegetables. Sometimes we ate beans instead or we just had meals without meat.

In 1955, right after high school, I moved to Washington, DC, and lived with my oldest sister, Manolia. She grew some of the same vegetables in her backyard that we had in the country. But at the time, I had no interest in helping her grow vegetables. It reminded me too much of the hard farm work back home.

I began to eat more fried and processed foods after I moved to DC, and within a few years, I started having chest pains. My doctor told me to cut back on fried foods, so I did somewhat, but not that much.

It wasn't until I was married and pregnant with my first child, Veronica, that I started reading about eating healthier. I wanted to find out how to have a healthy pregnancy and how to raise healthy children. This was in 1960 and Dr. Benjamin Spock's books on raising children were among the ones I read. By the time I had my second and third children, Marya and Tracye, a few years later, I was eating fewer fried and processed foods, but I still had a long way to go.

OVEREATING

When my girls were young, one weekend I decided to bake a three-layer German chocolate cake with coconut-pecan frosting. As it turned out, none of the girls liked the cake, and I ended up eating the entire thing by myself in two days. I got very sick and that's when I realized I had a problem with overeating. I had also been eating apple turnovers just about every day because the law firm where I worked had free pastries for breakfast. The first year I worked there I gained about ten pounds.

My sister, Ann, was already going to Overeaters Anonymous (OA), so I decided to start going with her. Everyone was surprised I was there because I wasn't overweight. But just because you're thin doesn't mean you're healthy.

When I found out there was an OA meeting near my office, I started going there during my lunch hour. At OA, I realized the reason I was overeating was that I was stressed. This was around 1970 and I was separated and bringing up my three children on my own. I was also dealing with racism at work as one of the first black employees at a majority white law firm. I realized that I was self-medicating with food to deal with the stress.

With OA's help, I was able to manage my overeating. In the process, I found out that it was harder to stop overeating foods that contain sugar, especially pastries and desserts, because sugar is addictive. So with OA's help, I also stopped eating sugar.

Then one day, after ten years had passed, I decided to eat a pastry. I figured that I had everything under control. But then one pastry led to another and after six months, I was back to being addicted to sugar. So I gave it up *again*. It was difficult at first—I was so addicted to sugar that I would often stand in front of a bakery just to smell the aroma. But the second time around, I was finally able to let it go completely. And still today, I don't knowingly eat anything that has refined sugar in it. I still eat desserts, but they're made with healthier sweeteners (as are the dessert recipes in this book).

HOW I WENT VEGAN

Letting go of sugar renewed my interest in learning more about healthy eating. And I read about several studies that came out linking pork and processed meat with an increased risk for cancer. So I decided to stop eating those foods, too.

Around that time, one of my brothers, Esau, died of a heart attack when he was in his fifties. And some of my cousins died of heart attacks soon after that, and they were also in their fifties. That's when I learned that red meat was linked to heart disease. I was forty-seven at the time and it was a real wake-up call. So I immediately stopped eating beef.

I also saw a documentary on how chicken was processed—about how they just cut off all the bad parts and sell the rest. So I threw out all the chicken in the freezer, and that was it for me with chicken.

By that time, Tracye was in college and was thinking about becoming a vegetarian, and she was encouraging me to go vegetarian, too. So I started reading all the books she had about it. I learned how harmful and polluted fish was, and I decided to let that go, too. So at that point, I had stopped eating all meat, but I was still eating cheese.

When I went for my annual physical, I told my doctor that I was a vegetarian and had given up everything but cheese. He said I should have given up cheese first because it had the most fat. So, that led me to eventually stop eating cheese. That was the hardest to give up! It took me about a year or so to do it. But once I made up my mind, I was able to let it go.

And that's how I went vegan at fifty. Looking back on it now, I know that giving up sugar first gave me the courage and strength to give up meat and dairy. I already knew I could do it.

MY BIGGEST CHALLENGES

In the beginning, being vegan was challenging in some ways because I had to learn about what to eat and how to prepare it. So I started experimenting with how to season beans and vegetables without meat. Tracye and I also experimented with cookbooks and recipes from the newspaper. This was in the late 1980s and early 1990s, before we had the Internet, so we didn't have as many resources available then. Fortunately, there were also vegan cafes close by, like Brown Rice and Soul Vegetarian, near Howard University. I also liked eating at Indian and Ethiopian restaurants because they had vegan dishes on the menu.

Being a vegan is effortless. It's just a natural part of who I am and I don't have to think about it. I know what to eat to stay healthy.

I think the most challenging part about being a vegan in those early years was going to restaurants with our extended family, where there were hardly any vegan options on the menu. Back in those days, it wasn't as easy to ask restaurants to prepare a vegan meal because they were so unfamiliar with veganism. So we usually just ate before or after we went to the restaurant. Or if we knew we were going to be at the restaurant for a few hours, we'd sometimes bring food with us, eat in the car, and then go in. We did what we had to do!

Every year we also have a big Thanksgiving dinner with our extended family and when we went vegan, we started to bring our own food, which we still do today. In the beginning, it was challenging because some of our relatives used to tease us with "What are you eating?" "Don't you want some chicken?" Some of my brothers, in particular, joked about it, but my sisters accepted it for the most part.

I remember when we went down to South Carolina to visit one of my older sisters and she said "Oh, you don't eat our food anymore?" That was hard. But then she prepared a huge pot of string beans and took a portion out for me before she put meat in it. So for my sisters, it wasn't that big of a deal. They always ate a lot of vegetables anyway.

My friends were the same way. They didn't have an issue with me becoming a vegan either. Maybe it had something to do with the fact that we were older. But they didn't treat me any differently because I wasn't eating the same things they were eating. When we ate out, we chose places where everyone could eat or we went to a vegetarian or vegan restaurant. Most of them liked the food, anyway.

Even at work, when food was served at meetings, there was never an issue. Just as I was a vegan, I had co-workers who ate kosher and other kinds of food. So the firm just provided different types of food. I didn't feel isolated at work in any way. In fact, at Christmas, I baked vegan cookies and my co-workers loved them.

CHANGES I EXPERIENCED AFTER GOING VEGAN

After I went vegan, people often commented that my skin looked good and had a healthy glow. I definitely noticed that, too. I think it's because I didn't eat a lot of processed vegan foods. There weren't that many vegan versions of meat and cheese available back then and I didn't like the way they tasted. I preferred to cook from scratch and eat whole foods. And I still prefer to eat that way today. It's one of the main reasons I've been able to stay healthy all these years.

Years ago, I also started growing fruits and vegetables in my backyard. I also had a community garden plot with Tracye and now I have one with Marya and my granddaughter, Mara. So I've come full circle.

Today, at eighty years old, I still don't have any chronic diseases, I'm not on any medications, and I'm not overweight. I weigh the same as I did in my thirties. I also exercise six days a week. I mainly take exercise classes at my senior center, usually twice a day. I do Pilates, aerobics, weight training, yoga, tai chi, and stretching and toning. Some of the other women in my exercise classes tell me I'm their inspiration. I love walking, too. Before I retired twenty years ago, I used to walk two miles in the mornings before going to work and at lunchtime. And, of course, I still walk today.

WHAT I LOVE ABOUT BEING A VEGAN

Being a vegan is effortless. It's just a natural part of who I am and I don't have to think about it. I know what to eat to stay healthy. And I'm healthy enough to do all the things I want to do and not feel any restrictions on my life. So I have the courage to try new things. I know that if I can bring up three children on my own, give up sugar, and go vegan, then I can do anything!

I know there are no guarantees when it comes to health. Things can happen through no fault of our own. But I also know that eating healthy vegan food gives me the best chance of maintaining good health. And as long as I live, I want to be as healthy as I can be so I can enjoy my life.

So when I tell people my age and they say things like "Oh, you look good! You don't look your age," I just tell them, "Well, how is an eighty-year-old supposed to look? Maybe this is it!"

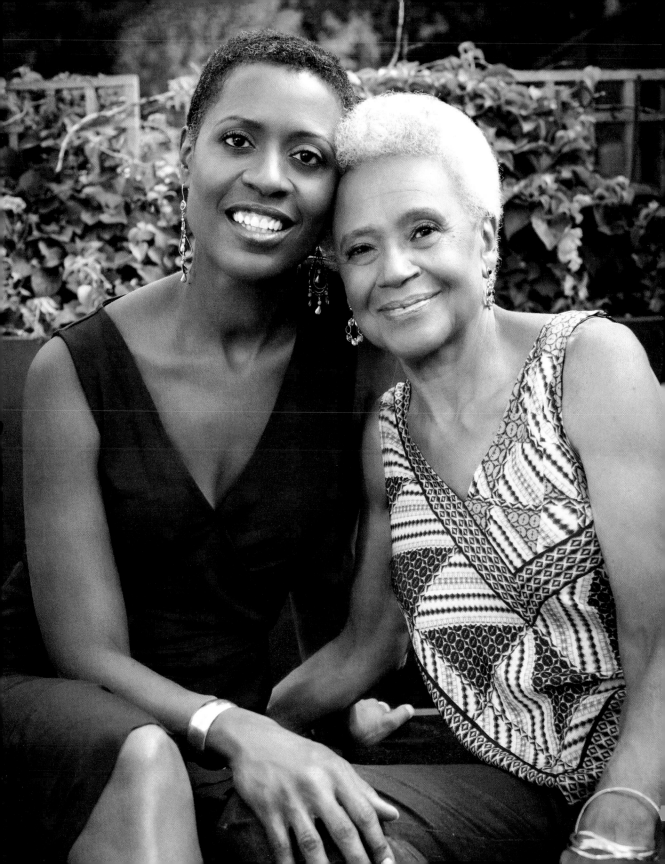

2

Eating for Health and Longevity

So now that you know why we became vegans, let's talk about the question we get asked the most: "What do you eat every day?" Well, the foods we eat each day are usually simple and wholesome. At this point in our vegan lives, we know exactly what to eat to maintain our health and vibrancy on a daily basis and for years to come—and it's pretty straightforward. In this chapter, we give you an easy set of guidelines that serve as the foundation for the way we eat and we tell you what a typical day of food looks like for us.

THE FAB FIVE FOOD RULES

We follow a few simple food principles when choosing what to eat each day. We call them our Fab Five Food Rules.

1. AT THE CORE.

We make sure to eat these central types of whole plant-based foods every day: fruits; vegetables; whole grains; and beans, nuts, and seeds. Creating our meals from these foods gives us unlimited ways to enjoy healthy, great-tasting dishes that meet all of our nutritional needs.

How much of the At the Core foods should you eat each day? Here's what that might look like for a moderately active woman (exercising up to 30 minutes daily) eating an average of 2,000 calories a day.

FRUITS 2 cups daily.

One cup is about the same as a piece of fruit, like a banana, orange, apple, grapefruit, or pear. It's also the same as a cup of blueberries, grapes, or strawberries (or about eight large strawberries) or a cup of chopped fruit. For dried fruits, like raisins and dried apricots, it's about a half cup each day.

VEGETABLES 2½ cups daily.

One cup is about the same as ten broccoli florets, twelve baby carrots, one large sweet potato, 1 cup of sliced beets, 1 cup of chopped zucchini, or 1 cup of sautéed collard greens. And 2 cups of raw, dark leafy greens are considered the equivalent of 1 cup of vegetables. (More on dark leafy greens, below.)

WHOLE GRAINS 1½ cups daily.

It's pretty easy to eat a cup and a half of cooked oatmeal, black rice, quinoa, millet, or whole-grain pasta each day. One slice of whole-grain bread or one whole-grain tortilla is also the equivalent of ½ cup of whole grains. So eating just one sandwich gets you two-thirds of the way to your daily recommended intake.

BEANS, NUTS, AND SEEDS 1½ cups of beans and ¼ cup of nuts daily.

Eating a cup and a half of beans each day could include a hot bowl of soup made from lentils, black beans, or split peas. And almonds, walnuts or cashews can be tossed into a morning smoothie.

2. KEEP YOUR BALANCE.

We create well-balanced meals. Whether in a breakfast smoothie, a lunch salad, or a dinner stir-fry, we make sure to eat a main source of protein (from beans or nuts), healthy fats (from nuts), and complex carbohydrates (from whole grains, vegetables, and fruits).

What does that look like in practice? For a typical 9-inch plate, you want to fill half with fruits and vegetables, one quarter with beans, and the other quarter with whole grains. Even with a wrap, burrito, or soup, you want to include fruits (remember, tomatoes are technically fruits), vegetables, whole grains, and beans.

3. HEALTH IS IN THE HUE.

We make sure our meals reflect the rainbow of colors in fruits, vegetables, whole grains, beans, and nuts. The colors or pigments in plant-based foods come from phytochemicals. These phytochemicals are protective compounds that provide numerous health benefits, from helping to prevent and reverse our major chronic diseases, including heart disease, cancer, stroke, and diabetes, to boosting our immune system and aiding in digestion. So the health is in the hue—and the darker and brighter the color, the greater the health benefits.

Want to get the health benefits of the food rainbow each day? Well, you're probably already eating at least some brightly colored foods every day. An orange, tomatoes, carrots? Just start upping your game by including at least two to three bright colors at each meal, from red beans to purple eggplant, to yellow squash. (See more suggestions for colorful food in chapter 3).

4. BY ANY GREENS NECESSARY.

We eat dark leafy greens two to three times a day. They provide the most nutrition of all foods and have the fewest calories. In fact, they have so many health benefits that researchers have yet to discover them all. But we do know that the phytochemicals, vitamins, and minerals in dark leafy greens protect against heart disease, cancer, and stroke, as well as improve memory and vision and help build strong bones. My mother and I each eat about one standard bunch of greens or twelve to fifteen leaves per day. This is one of the keys to our health and longevity, in addition to eating whole foods.

Want to stay ageless, too? Try to eat at least 4 cups of dark leafy greens every day. It's not as hard as you might think. Here's what that might look like:

MORNING DRINK Add 1 to 2 cups of fresh or frozen spinach or kale to a fruit smoothie.

LUNCH Have 2 cups of kale, arugula, dandelion greens, or other combination of dark leafy greens be the foundation of your salad.

DINNER Add very thinly chopped chard as a garnish to the other types of vegetables you have for dinner.

5. SMALL IS ALL.

We eat four to five small meals throughout the day, rather than three large meals. This helps us maintain our energy levels and leads to better absorption of nutrients that our bodies can use throughout the day.

Want to eat smaller meals throughout the day without going hungry? Focus on quality over quantity. Here's what that might look like:

MORNING Green smoothie

MID-MORNING Oatmeal with nuts and fruit

LUNCH Soup and salad

MID-AFTERNOON Hummus and avocado with whole-grain crackers

DINNER Vegetable wrap or veggie pizza.

EVERYDAY EATS

With these Fab Five Food Rules as our foundation, here's what we eat every day.

TRACYE

MORNING

I drink a glass of water first thing in the morning around 7:00 a.m. Then I blend dandelion greens with water and freshly squeezed lemon juice in a high-speed blender and drink 2 cups. This drink is not only nutrient-rich, it makes me feel calm and mellow, and helps my skin maintain its healthy glow.

After I exercise, around 8:00 a.m., I drink a green smoothie made with water; a cup of fresh or frozen dark leafy greens (usually dandelion greens, spinach, collards, or kale); a cup of fresh or frozen berries (I switch up between blueberries, blackberries, raspberries, strawberries, and others); a banana or avocado for creaminess; fresh ginger; and hemp seeds. Sometimes I'll swap out the hemp seeds for half a cup of nuts or 2 tablespoons of ground flaxseed meal. (See part 2 for the Liquid Sunshine Dandelion Lemon Drink and Tracye's Daily Green Smoothie recipes.)

MID-MORNING

I usually eat a bowl of oatmeal by 11:00 a.m., using rolled oats, a chopped apple, a handful of walnuts, and a dash of cinnamon. I might also swap a teaspoon or two of chia seeds (which are high in omega-3 fatty acids) for the walnuts.

AFTERNOON

For lunch, I may have a sprouted whole-grain wrap with either black beans, lentils, pinto beans, chickpeas, or other beans, along with multicolored bell peppers, mushrooms, black olives, avocados, shredded purple cabbage and carrots, chopped kale, garlic, and red onions. Or I may have a bowl of bean soup or oven-grilled tofu or tempeh with a kale salad. (See part 2 for the Pinto Bean Wrap, Crispy Tofu Bites, and All Hail the Kale Salad Remix recipes.)

MID-AFTERNOON

A few hours after lunch, I may have red bell pepper hummus with nori sheets or whole-grain crackers and one or two pieces of fruit, like an orange, mango, peach, or persimmon (depending on the season). I'll also have green tea or chamomile tea.

EVENING

Dinner is often a lightly sautéed dish. This could be sautéed collards with pine nuts, mushrooms, sun-dried tomatoes, and garlic over whole-grain pasta, black rice, or curry quinoa. Or it could be string beans or broccoli, multicolored bell peppers, mushrooms, corn, and nuts with a creamy sauce over one of the whole grains above. (See part 2 for the Collards and Quinoa, String Beans with Shiitake Mushrooms and Almonds, and Vegetable Stir-Fry with Black Rice and Almond Butter Sauce recipes.)

WATER

Along with my morning water, dandelion greens drink, green smoothie, and tea, I typically drink four to five more glasses of water throughout the day. The raw fruit and vegetables I eat also have a high water content.

MARY

MORNING AND MID-MORNING

The first thing I do in the morning is drink one glass of plain water and then one glass of water with juice from half of a large lemon and one-fourth teaspoon of cayenne pepper. If I have an 8:00 a.m. exercise class, before I go I'll have a smoothie made with water, a half-cup of blueberries, an apple, two cups of chopped fresh kale, freshly squeezed lemon juice, two tablespoons of flax seeds, and I may add in three tablespoons of hemp protein powder. This makes about one-and-a-half cups. (See part 2 for Mary's Daily Green Smoothie recipe.)

Then after class, around 10:00 a.m., I'll eat a bowl of oatmeal made with rolled oats, a half-cup of walnuts, and a half-cup of raisins or one date.

Or on mornings that I have a 9:00 a.m. exercise class, I'll eat a bowl of oatmeal instead of having a smoothie. With the oatmeal, I'll have nutritional yeast, almonds, chia seeds, turmeric, and cumin. Sometimes I'll add chopped raw kale, as well. This makes a filling breakfast that will leave me feeling satisfied for a few hours.

Then after that, I'll make one-and-a-half cups of green drink. I blend dark leafy greens, like kale, spinach, collards, beet greens, or dandelion greens with water in a blender.

AFTERNOON

For lunch, I may have black bean soup or three-bean soup with carrots, onions, garlic, sweet potatoes, and celery. I'll also have a dandelion greens salad with chopped avocado, onion, and garlic. I usually don't put salad dressing on it. I may just place the hot beans on top, which softens the greens. Sometimes I'll eat whole-grain crackers with the soup and salad or I'll have a baked sweet potato instead of the crackers. (See part 2 for the Three-Bean Chili and Citrusy Dandelion Greens Salad recipes.)

Or instead of soup, I may have a black bean burger and use kale or collards instead of lettuce. I usually eat sprouted whole-grain bread with the burger, but sometimes I'll use collard leaves and eat it like a pita.

MID-AFTERNOON

I usually have fresh fruit, like an apple, banana, peach, grapes, cherries, or cantaloupe (depending on the season) or I'll have apricots, figs, or dates.

EVENING

For dinner, I may have a stir-fry with tempeh or tofu, broccoli, onions, and garlic. I'll have that with quinoa and a kale salad with avocado, a little olive oil, and garlic.

Or I may have a curried chickpea salad along with brown rice or millet and roasted red and yellow peppers. With that, I may have roasted Brussels sprouts or roasted cauliflower. (See part 2 for the Curried Chickpeas in Warm Pita Pocket, Balsamic Brussels Sprouts, and Roasted Curried Cauliflower recipes.)

WATER

I try to drink at least six cups of water daily, which includes the two glasses I drink in the early morning, as well as two cups of herbal tea, particularly green tea. The other two are plain glasses of water I drink during the day. During the summer, I usually drink more water, especially with my daily exercises.

Overall, we keep our meals light, nutritious, and delicious. With the Fab Five Food Rules, you can easily put this into practice in your own life based on your own tastes, preferences, and circumstances.

THE PROTEIN QUESTION

The other most common question we get is, "How do you get enough protein?" First, rest assured that it's easy to get more than enough protein from plant-based foods. In fact, the largest study in history of people who eat plant-based diets, published in the *Journal of the Academy of Nutrition and Dietetics* in 2013, found that the average vegan gets 70 percent more protein than the recommended daily allowance—just like meat-eaters do.

But just what is that daily allowance? On average, we need to get about 50–70 grams a day, according to the Institute of Medicine. Another way to calculate that is to multiply your weight by 0.36 grams. So if you're 140 pounds, you'll need about 50 grams of protein each day. If you're very physically active, you need more protein, up to 70 grams daily, and you can easily meet your needs by increasing the amount of protein-rich beans, nuts, and grains you eat each day from the list below.

TOP TEN HIGH-PROTEIN VEGAN FOODS

1. **TEMPEH**, ½ 8-ounce package = 22 grams (See chapter 3 for more on tempeh)
2. **TOFU**, 1 cup cooked = 20 grams
3. **LENTILS**, 1 cup cooked = 18 grams
4. **PUMPKIN SEEDS**, ½ cup raw = 17 grams
5. **ALMONDS**, ½ cup raw = 16 grams
6. **SPLIT PEAS**, 1 cup cooked = 16 grams
7. **CHICKPEAS (GARBANZO BEANS)**, 1 cup cooked = 15 grams (most beans have 14–16 grams per cup cooked)
8. **PISTACHIOS**, ½ cup raw = 12.5 grams
9. **HEMP SEEDS (HEMP HEARTS)**, ¼ cup raw (4 tablespoons) = 10 grams
10. **QUINOA**, 1 cup cooked = 9 grams

Keep in mind that almost all plant-based foods contain some amount of protein, from an avocado (7 grams) to a cup of raw kale (2 grams). The key is to eat different plant-based foods throughout the day, and you'll easily meet all of your protein needs.

What About Vitamin B₁₂?

Vitamin B_{12} originates from bacteria, not plants or animals. It's made by tiny one-celled organisms or microbes that are in the earth and water. As Dr. Michael Greger details in *How Not to Die*, the latest research findings show the healthiest and most reliable plant-based sources of vitamin B_{12} in our diets are B_{12}-fortified foods, including breakfast cereals, plant-based milks, and nutritional yeast (see description on page 56) or B_{12} supplements.

It really is simple to eat healthy, well-balanced, vegan meals on a daily basis. In the next chapter, we talk about superfoods you can add to your plate to help keep you ageless.

SUPERFOODS THAT KEEP YOU GLOWING

It's never too early or too late to start eating for better health and longevity. The foods you eat today—whether you're in your twenties, forties, sixties, eighties or beyond—will help determine how healthy you'll be in the future and how long a future you've got. In fact, as we get older, our health doesn't have to decline from chronic diseases, and our bodies don't have to deteriorate. It's actually normal to be healthy and disease-free as we get older. And eating whole plant-based foods is the key.

Plant-based foods contain high amounts of antioxidants, which are powerful compounds that can slow down the aging process by protecting cells from oxidative stress. Oxidative stress—often referred to as rusting of the cells—can be caused by the effects of internal factors, like harmful free radicals, and by the effects of external factors, like harmful lifestyle, and environmental and societal conditions (unhealthy foods, pollution, and racism are examples). This oxidative stress on the cellular level contributes to the conditions most commonly associated with aging: cognitive decline and memory loss, skin wrinkling, bone and muscle weakening, and vision loss and impairment.

But the antioxidants in plant-based foods can help counter these conditions. Some plant-based foods are much higher in antioxidants than others and so have more anti-aging benefits. These foods are called superfoods because they're especially beneficial for long-term health and well-being. The most antioxidant-rich superfoods are deeply colored fruits, vegetables, herbs, and spices.

Here's a list of twenty-two anti-aging superfoods that can improve the health of your brain, skin, bones, muscles, and eyes that are also featured in the recipes in this book.

FOODS THAT PROMOTE BRAIN POWER

BLUEBERRIES AND STRAWBERRIES

These berries contain anthocyanidins, which are health-promoting plant pigments that give certain fruits and vegetables their rich blue, red, and purple colors. Research from the Nurses' Health Study has shown that these compounds in blueberries and strawberries can help improve brain functioning as we get older by concentrating in areas of the brain involved with memory and learning. Eating a total of 1 cup of blueberries and 2 cups of strawberries each week has been shown to slow cognitive decline in older women by as much as two and a half years.

BLUEBERRY RECIPES

Tracye's Daily Green Smoothie
(page 62)

Mary's Daily Green Smoothie
(page 63)

Chia Berry Breakfast Pudding
(page 88)

Sunrise Smoothie Bowl (page 87)

Blueberry Muffins (page 93)

STRAWBERRY RECIPES

Berry Beet Smoothie (page 70)

Maple French Toast with Strawberries
(page 98)

Sunrise Smoothie Bowl (page 87)

Fruity Ice Pops (page 225)

CELERY

As a rich source of an antioxidant and anti-inflammatory plant compound called luteolin, celery helps protect against brain inflammation that can lead to dementia. Aim to add a serving of celery to your meals two to three times a week. One serving is about 1 cup of chopped celery or two 10-inch celery stalks.

RECIPES

Lemongrass Noodle Soup (page 125)

Curried Lentil Soup with Carrots and Rosemary (page 130)

Farro with Shiitake Mushrooms (page 123)

Three-Bean Chili (page 204)

ROSEMARY

This aromatic herb has been shown to improve memory and brain function. As an evergreen, low-maintenance plant, rosemary is one of the easiest herbs to grow yourself, making it simple and convenient to sprinkle fresh or dried leaves on your meals throughout the week.

RECIPES

Curried Lentil Soup with Carrots and Rosemary (page 130)

Roasted Beet Slices with Rosemary (page 163)

Roasted Root Vegetables (page 157)

SAFFRON

This distinctive crimson spice from the *Crocus sativus* flower has been shown to diminish the cognition-impairing effects of mild to moderate Alzheimer's disease. Saffron is one of the world's most expensive spices to produce, but fortunately a few pinches are typically all you need to reap the health benefits of cooking with it, especially when adding it to whole grains.

RECIPE
Saffron Rice (page 131)

TURMERIC

This powerful orange spice has been used in Southeast Asian cuisines for thousands of years. Turmeric has been shown to help prevent Alzheimer's disease or reduce its symptoms, among its many other health benefits. In fact, because of its effectiveness in the prevention and treatment of a wide range of health conditions, turmeric is one of the few spices that should be consumed daily. In *How Not to Die*, Dr. Michael Greger recommends consuming ¼ teaspoon of turmeric each day. And be sure to use turmeric with a pinch of black pepper to dramatically increase its effectiveness.

RECIPES
Curried Tofu Scramble with Shiitake Mushrooms (page 101)
Crunchy Roasted Chickpeas (page 106)
Crispy Tofu Bites (page 111)
Thai Coconut Curry Soup (page 120)
Curried Lentil Soup with Carrots and Rosemary (page 130)
Chana Masala (page 141)
Mac and Cheese (page 142)
Ethiopian Platter (page 202)
Collards and Quinoa (page 165)
Roasted Curried Cauliflower (page 168)

FOODS THAT HELP SKIN STAY SMOOTH

CORN AND PEAS

A 2010 study published in the *British Journal of Nutrition* found that the beta carotene in yellow and green vegetables like corn and peas can help reduce facial wrinkling around the eyes, also known as crow's feet.

CORN RECIPES
Home-Style Grits (page 100)
Avocado Quesadillas with Salsa and Cashew Sour Cream (page 102)
Southern-Style Cornbread (page 128)
Enchiladas (page 189)
Roasted Sweet Potato and Black Bean Bowl with
  Lime Cilantro Vinaigrette (page 194)
Vegetable Pot Pie (page 199)
Black-Eyed Peas Salad (page 137)

Roasted Corn on the Cob with Spicy Rub (page 156)

Rainbow Slaw (page 167)

PEA RECIPES
Sweet Pea Hummus (page 114)

Vegetable Pot Pie (page 199)

FLAXSEEDS, CHIA SEEDS, HEMP SEEDS, AND WALNUTS

The omega-3 fatty acids in these seeds and nuts have been found to help prevent premature wrinkling of the skin. Be sure to use ground flaxseed meal for easier digestion. A serving of ground flaxseed meal and chia seeds is 2 tablespoons each. A serving of hemp seeds is 4 tablespoons, and a serving of walnuts is ¼ cup.

FLAXSEED RECIPES
Mary's Daily Green Smoothie
   (page 63)

Blueberry Muffins (page 93)

Perfect Pecan Pie (page 217)

Fudge Walnut Brownies (page 212)

Pineapple Carrot Cupcakes with
   Orange Cashew Cream Topping
   (page 226)

CHIA SEED RECIPES
Chia Berry Breakfast Pudding
   (page 88)

Sunrise Smoothie Bowl (page 87)

HEMP SEED RECIPES
Tracye's Daily Green Smoothie
   (page 62)

WALNUT RECIPES
Sweet Potato Smoothie (page 68)

Banana Walnut Muffins (page 91)

Stuffed Orange and Red Bell Peppers (page 186)

Arugula Salad with Walnuts and Caesar Dressing (page 148)

Swiss Chard Sauté with Walnuts (page 152)

Hazelnut Date Bars (page 213)

Fudge Walnut Brownies (page 212)

Pineapple Carrot Cupcakes with Orange Cashew Cream Topping (page 226)

GREEN TEA

Sipping this tea has been shown to delay the appearance of wrinkles and expression lines, as well as improve skin hydration and elasticity and improve overall skin quality.

RECIPE
Green Tea with Ginger and Cardamom (page 74)

KIWI

This fuzzy fruit is exceptionally high in vitamin C, which helps to maintain the collagen and elastin essential for firm skin. One large kiwi has enough vitamin C to meet the daily requirement.

RECIPES
Watermelon Kiwi Lime Smoothie (page 69)
Fruity Ice Pops (page 225)
Almost Ambrosia (page 229)

FOODS THAT STRENGTHEN BONES AND MUSCLES

KALE AND SWISS CHARD

These dark leafy greens are exceptionally high in vitamin K, which helps promote bone strength and increase bone density. One cup of each (raw or cooked) exceeds the daily requirement by more than three times. Beet greens, collards, mustards, and spinach are also excellent sources of vitamin K.

KALE RECIPES
Tracye's Daily Green Smoothie (page 62)
Mary's Daily Green Smoothie (page 63)
Navy Bean and Kale Soup (page 127)
Pinto Bean Wrap (page 177)
All Hail the Kale Salad Remix (page 160)
Braised Sesame Kale (page 166)

SWISS CHARD RECIPE
Swiss Chard Sauté with Walnuts (page 152)

SWEET POTATOES

This root vegetable is high in potassium (nearly twice as high as a banana), and potassium has been shown to help improve muscle strength and protect bone health.

RECIPES
Sweet Potato Smoothie (page 68)
Spiced and Sautéed Sweet Potatoes (page 136)
Baked Sweet Potato Fries with Garlic and Truffle Oil (page 133)
Roasted Sweet Potato and Black Bean Bowl with
  Lime Cilantro Vinaigrette (page 194)
Roasted Root Vegetables (page 157)

FOODS THAT IMPROVE VISION

KALE, SPINACH, BROCCOLI, AND CORN

In *Never Too Late to Go Vegan*, authors Carol J. Adams, Patti Breitman, and Virginia Messina, MPH, RD, encourage the consumption of kale, spinach, broccoli, and corn for maintaining good vision as we age. These vegetables are high in lutein and zeaxanthin, which are antioxidants that are deposited in the macula, the central area of the eye's retina. These antioxidants filter out UV rays and harmful free radicals to help prevent cataracts and macular degeneration that can lead to vision loss. In addition, a 2011 study published in the *American Journal of Clinical Nutrition* of more than twenty-seven thousand people over age forty found that vegans had a 40 percent lower chance of getting cataracts than omnivores, which was associated with their higher intake of fruit and vegetables.

KALE RECIPES
See Kale Recipes under Foods That Strengthen Bones and Muscles

SPINACH RECIPES
Pineapple Spinach Smoothie (page 64)
Artichoke Dip with Pita Chips (page 112)
Savory Vegetable Quiche (page 200)
Lasagna with Mushrooms, Eggplant, and Zucchini (page 188)

BROCCOLI RECIPES
Thai Coconut Curry Soup (page 120)
Lemongrass Noodle Soup (page 125)
Pad Thai (page 180)
Vegetable Stir-Fry with Black Rice and Almond Butter Sauce (page 192)

CORN RECIPES
See Corn Recipes under Foods That Help Skin Stay Smooth

CARROTS

The high beta carotene content of carrots converts to vitamin A in the body and helps to improve vision function, especially night vision. Beta carotene also helps protect skin from harmful UV radiation from the sun.

RECIPES
Summer Rolls (page 115)
Yellow Split Pea Soup with Red Onion (page 122)
Thai Coconut Curry Soup (page 120)

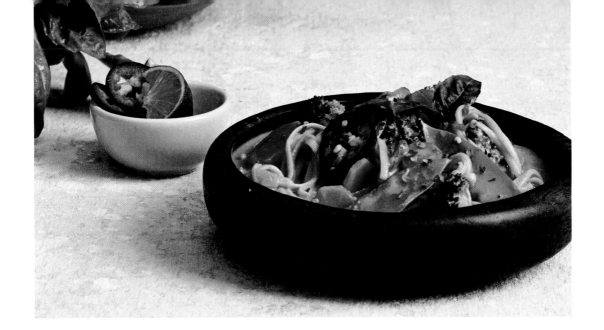

Lemongrass Noodle Soup (page 125)

Curried Lentil Soup with Carrots and Rosemary (page 130)

Pad Thai (page 180)

Buckwheat Soba Bowl (page 182)

Black Bean Soup with Avocado and Cashew Sour Cream (page 144)

Purple Cabbage Bowl (page 174)

Vegetable Pot Pie (page 199)

Ethiopian Platter (page 202)

Three-Bean Chili (page 204)

Roasted Root Vegetables (page 157)

All Hail the Kale Salad Remix (page 160)

Rainbow Slaw (page 167)

Pineapple Carrot Cupcakes with Orange Cashew Cream Topping (page 226)

This list will help you get started eating more anti-aging foods. Keep in mind that you don't have to eat these foods every day to reap their anti-aging benefits. Strive to rotate some of these foods on your plate each week. The most important thing to remember is that eating a wide variety of fruits, vegetables, herbs, and spices each day will give you an abundance of antioxidants you need to grow older healthfully. And because these foods have the added bonus of decreasing your risk of chronic diseases, they'll help you live longer, too.

The recipes in this book are helpfully coded (see page 59) when they include these superfood ingredients and when they reflect some of our Fab Five Food Rules.

FOURTEEN STEPS TO A HEALTHIER YOU

We know that going vegan for the long term might seem challenging, but don't worry. We've been there, so here are fourteen steps to help you transition to a healthier lifestyle with ease and grace—and to help you eat even healthier if you're already a vegan. This guide offers tried-and-true recommendations based on what we've done to stay vibrantly vegan for decades and have taught others to do, as well. These steps will make it easier for you, too, to become an ageless vegan.

1. Know Your Why
2. Liberate Your Mind and Your Mouth Will Follow
3. Choose a Date and Begin
4. Find Your People
5. Know That You're Worth It
6. Start Where You Are
7. Eat Whole Foods
8. Explore New Recipes
9. Plan Your Meals
10. Read the Label
11. Stay on Budget
12. Eat Out with Ease
13. Keep a Stash
14. Enjoy the Journey

STEP 1: KNOW YOUR WHY

The focus of step 1 is to get clear about why you want to go vegan. Is it for your health, the animals, the environment, social justice, spirituality, faith, or other reasons? Your why often comes as a reaction to something you've watched, like a documentary about factory farming or global warming. Or conversations you've had with a friend or family member who's vegan. Or a book you've read about someone's transition story or about how to go vegan. Or a flash of insight you have about animals while eating a piece of meat or even playing with your dog. Or it could be a personal health crisis that you or a loved one is experiencing that ultimately leads you to change the way you eat.

Whatever the reason is, be sure you're passionate about it. Be sure you understand it and believe it. This foundation is crucial because as you begin your transition, there will be inevitable obstacles along the way. For example, the meat and dairy you used to eat will probably still look and smell good to you—especially during the first few weeks or months of your transition. And eating differently than many of your friends or people in your family, community, or culture may be emotionally and socially challenging for you in the beginning.

Being confident in why you're going vegan will help you overcome these challenges. To help you get there, write down your reason for making the transition. Write it on sticky notes or beautiful notecards and place them on your bedroom mirror, on your refrigerator, on your kitchen counter, in your wallet, in your car, on your desk at work—you get the picture. All of these notes will remind you of your why, your intention, your purpose for going vegan. It will be inspiration and affirmation just when you need it most.

Continue to learn more about veganism and that knowledge will also help you know your why, as we'll discuss in step 2. Just know that once you've truly embraced your why, you'll be at peace with your choice.

STEP 2: LIBERATE YOUR MIND AND YOUR MOUTH WILL FOLLOW

Step 2 is to continuously learn about veganism, especially the aspect of it that you're most passionate about. Read and watch all that you can to stay informed. And talk to vegans about what they love most about their vegan lifestyle, how they transitioned, what challenges they faced, and how they overcame them.

Supporting yourself with knowledge is key. An informal 2013 online survey of more than seven thousand vegans conducted by The Vegan Truth blog found that more than 40 percent of respondents were inspired to go vegan after watching an educational video or movie; nearly 30 percent were motivated by an article, book, or song lyric; and another 25 percent were encouraged to become vegans after a conversation with another person.

Also, as I mentioned in chapter 1, after Dick Gregory's fateful lecture, I read everything I could find about vegetarianism and decided to go vegetarian, then vegan, as a result. I still have that same passion for learning today (even after getting a master's degree in public health nutrition). There's always new research being done that can help me tweak the way I eat to stay healthy. In fact, the nonprofit website NutritionFacts.org is one of my favorite sites to find out about the latest in nutrition research. I encourage you to check it out, if you haven't already. I also urge you to identify other go-to resources that focus on *your* particular reason for going vegan.

Staying up on the latest vegan information will also help you answer those persistent questions from vegan-curious folks and naysayers. You can practice short, to-the-point answers to common questions like "Where do you get your protein?" with quick facts like the one mentioned in chapter 2: "Vegans get 70 percent more protein than the recommended daily allowance—just like meat-eaters do." Or you can simply refer them to your favorite fact-based films, books, or websites to explore for themselves, just like you did.

STEP 3: CHOOSE A DATE AND BEGIN

Once you've decided you want to go vegan, setting a specific start date will help you make your intention a reality. It will give you a concrete goal to look forward to and work toward.

When choosing a start date, I suggest picking one that's in the very near future, about two weeks to two months away. You don't want to choose a date too much farther than that because you could lose your momentum and begin to doubt your decision. But you also don't want a date that's too close, like tomorrow or next Monday, because it may not give you enough time to prepare to make the transition—which could include restocking your kitchen (see chapter 3).

I also recommend choosing a date that doesn't have a separate, special significance, like your birthday, an anniversary, or even New Year's Day. Those days may bring up emotions (whether pleasant or unpleasant) that crowd out your desire to transition. And if celebration food is involved, you may be tempted to "just have a little" or overindulge in the very foods you want to avoid.

You could choose instead to transition on a national or international holiday dedicated to eating vegan foods or one that is vegan-related, like The Great American Meatout on March 20, Earth Day on April 22, World Vegetarian Day on October 1, or World Vegan Day on November 1.

Or you can make your transition date its own special day by celebrating it with a fabulous vegan meal with friends and family. You could also just pick a random date that reflects your everyday life to symbolize the normalcy with which you'll incorporate being vegan into your lifestyle.

So however you choose to recognize it, choose a start date, mark it on your calendar, and make your goal a reality.

STEP 4: FIND YOUR PEOPLE

Now more than ever, there's no need to start your vegan journey alone. First look to your inner circle for support: your family and closest friends. If some of them are already vegan, are going vegan, or are otherwise very supportive, that's wonderful! Be grateful to have a built-in support system (just as my family did). It can make a world of difference.

But what if your family and friends aren't supportive? And what if you not only want their support, but you want them to go vegan with you? Well, I encourage you to focus first on yourself and be an example. As a new vegan, of course you want your loved ones to know how healthy plant foods are; how unhealthy animal foods are; how terrible conditions are for chickens, cow, and pigs on factory farms; how harmful factory farming is for people and the planet; the inequity of our current food system; and more.

But even with all that urgency, first be an example. If your loved ones ask about veganism, then cook vegan food with them, visit vegan restaurants together, and talk, watch films, read books, and go to vegan events together. If they want to learn more for themselves and be supportive of you, that's great. If they don't, continue on your vegan journey and let things flow organically.

You can also seek out support by joining your local vegan Meetup group. Meetups are a great way to meet people who are newly vegan, experienced vegans, or vegan-friendly. And you'll meet people who are interested in veganism for a variety of reasons that may be different from your own. Of if there's no vegan Meetup in your area, consider starting one. You might be surprised at how many like-minded people you can help bring together to share in vegan activities.

And know that all your activities with other vegans don't have to be vegan-related. In fact, one of the joys of just being in places where vegan and vegan-friendly people are in the majority is that veganism is the given, the norm. So you can just be yourself and not have veganism be the main topic of conversation.

For example, my family has been going to the annual Vegetarian Society of Washington, DC, vegan Thanksgiving gala for years. But beyond the vegan-focused keynote address, veganism is not what we chat about with our friends. It's a completely different experience from being "the vegan" at other holiday gatherings. Worrying about the food and being peppered with questions about being vegan can put a damper on the festivities.

So that's why it's good to be where the vegans are if you want to be vegan. Seek out environments where being vegan is just regular, natural, a nonissue. Like your local vegan group or an online vegan community. Spend some quality time with your people. That's how you get the support you need and make being vegan your new normal.

STEP 5: KNOW THAT YOU'RE WORTH IT

This is a step that I thought a lot about before adding. I didn't want to suggest that if people don't go vegan, then somehow they don't have self-worth. So just to be clear, that's not what I'm saying here at all.

What I *am* saying is that if you want to go vegan, but you're letting fear of what other people might think or fear of doing something that most people you know and love aren't doing (even after reading step 4 for help with this), I understand that this is a real concern. I know that this anxiety has kept many people from going vegan. So that's why I'm including it in these fourteen steps. Because I want you to know that if going vegan is something that you want to do, you can do it because intrinsically you're worth it.

Let me share a story with you. Back in 2001, I was going to graduate school at NYU for my master's degree in public health nutrition. At that point, I had been vegan for about thirteen years. One day I was waiting for a friend at her office and started chatting with her co-worker, whom I had talked to several times before.

This particular time, we talked about my veganism. I'm not sure how the topic came up, because I don't usually bring it up in casual conversation. But for whatever reason, we were talking about it. He was a staunch meat-eater and couldn't understand why I'd want to be a vegan. And one of the questions he asked me was "How can you do something that no one else is doing?" And what struck me was the *way* he asked it, as if the fact that most people weren't vegan automatically called into question the legitimacy of being vegan. It was the first time I can remember someone using that as a rationale.

And I remember looking at him incredulously, wondering how he could think that way. As an activist, my immediate reaction had to do with the premise of his question—that of doing something counter to society. My thought was that we're both black, and if we're both critical thinkers and just have plain common sense, we know that most of what we do for our own benefit, health, and happiness already runs counter to this society's systemic white supremacy. And for black women, it runs counter to society's systemic white supremacist patriarchy. So that alone made his question perplexing to me.

I also knew that just because most people weren't doing something was not a reason *not* to do something that's good for me. The fact that I wanted to do it was enough. I had to follow my path. And as it turned out, I got a lot of support from my family and community, for which I was thankful. I would not have experienced that if I'd waited for everyone else to go vegan first. In fact, I'd still be waiting thirty years later! And I would have missed the opportunity to help so many people live healthier lives and to help expand this vegan movement over the last three decades.

So with that said, I urge you to follow that whisper or shout from within that's saying "I want to go vegan." You're worthy of listening to that voice. And you're worthy of doing what's healthiest for you. You don't have to wait for most people to do it. That may or may not happen. But *you* can start now. You're already worth it. And you never know how many people you'll inspire along the way!

STEP 6: START WHERE YOU ARE

Starting where you are means taking a closer look at the food you're already eating on a regular basis. First, do this exercise: write down what you typically eat Monday through Friday for breakfast, lunch, and dinner. It should include the meat and dairy that you may normally eat. Your list doesn't have to be exact—just write five breakfasts, five lunches, and five dinners that you might eat in any given week.

Now see if any of the meals on your list are already vegan. For example, do you have a smoothie or cereal or oatmeal with almond milk or soy milk for breakfast? For lunch, do you have a veggie wrap or a side salad with a vinaigrette or balsamic dressing? For dinner, do you have pasta with marinara sauce? Are there any other typical meals that come to mind that might already be vegan?

Along these same lines, also remember that most, if not all, of the herbs and spices you probably season your food with are already vegan. They're just fresh, dried, or powdered plants. The liquid seasonings you may use, like hot sauce, barbecue sauce, and soy sauce, are also typically vegan. The same is also true for the olive oil, sesame oil, or generic vegetable oil you may use. And the flour you may use is also vegan, although if it's white flour, you'll want to swap it out for a healthier, whole-grain flour (see step 7).

Next, look at how you can easily veganize most of the meals on your list that have meat and dairy. If you eat dairy yogurt for breakfast, you can switch to nondairy yogurt made with coconut, cashew, hemp seed, almond, or other plant-based milk. For lunch, you can swap out a beef burrito for a spicy bean burrito with guacamole and salsa, or with nondairy cheese, if you'd prefer. For dinner, instead of a chicken and veggie stir-fry, you can have a colorful vegetable stir-fry with almonds over wild rice. You'll be surprised at how easily you can make your most familiar meals vegan.

Finally, starting where you are also applies to folks who are already vegan or vegetarian. There's probably one thing you know you can do to up your game and take your health to the next level. If you're a vegetarian, it may be letting go of dairy products. If you're a vegan, it may be eating a more balanced diet that includes more dark-green leafy vegetables and whole grains. You can do the same exercise: write out a week's worth of meals, and see where you can make healthier changes. Whatever it is for you, you can get started today.

STEP 7: EAT WHOLE FOODS

As I mentioned in chapter 1, the central types of vegan foods are fruits, vegetables, whole grains, beans, nuts, and seeds. From these categories, you can easily create an infinite variety of nutritious and delicious meals that meet all of your nutritional needs.

So when I talk about eating whole foods, I mean eating these foods closest to their natural, unprocessed, nutrient-rich state. For whole grains, that means black, brown, or wild rice; quinoa; oats; barley; millet; amaranth; and more. These whole grains contain an abundance of vitamins, minerals, and essential fiber.

Fiber, in particular, helps to prevent plaque from building up in your arteries, decreasing your risk for heart attack and stroke. Fiber also helps maintain a steady blood sugar level, which reduces your risk for diabetes. And fiber protects against other diseases, including obesity and cancer, as well as diverticulosis and constipation.

On the other hand, processed or refined grains, like white rice, white pasta, white bread, and bakery products made with white flour have had most of the fiber, vitamins, and minerals removed. Manufacturers then add in a few synthetic nutrients and call it "enriched," a true oxymoron. These nutrient-deficient grains are quite harmful and can increase your risk for heart disease, diabetes, and obesity.

So remember, just because it's vegan, doesn't mean it's healthy. This also applies to processed packaged foods, especially those designed to mimic the look, texture, and taste of meat and dairy products. These are what I call bridge or transitional foods. They may help you cross over from omnivore to vegan, but they're not a place to stay. They're typically higher in fat, salt, and sugar. So they may be healthier than meat and dairy, but they're not necessarily healthy.

Your best bet is to center your meals on whole foods. You'll have an abundance of nutritious and great-tasting vegan foods available to you, as you'll see with the whole-food recipes in this book.

STEP 8: EXPLORE NEW RECIPES

In addition to eating your way through our delicious recipes, you'll want to continuously try new recipes. This is key in the beginning, as you learn your way around new vegan foods. The fact is, once vegan foods become your new normal, you'll probably get bored with your food from time to time, just like you did as an omnivore. So getting into the habit of exploring new recipes now will help you move through those periods more easily.

You can start by browsing vegan recipe sites once a week and bookmarking or pinning the recipes you'd like to try. These recipes will become your new favorites for inspiration at meal-planning time. You can also check out vegan cookbooks and magazines at libraries and bookstores to expand your awareness about the wide variety of vegan dishes possible. And it'll help to make vegan meals the default in your mind when it comes to food.

Taking food preparation classes is another great way to try new recipes when you're transitioning to vegan foods. You may need to learn a whole new

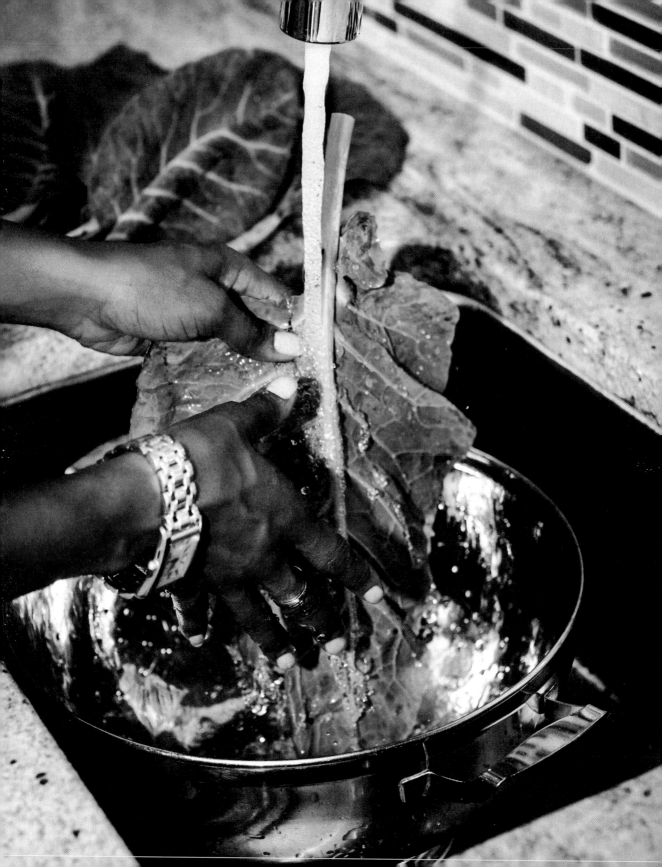

set of skills. Taking classes from an expert in vegan cooking is an ideal way to shorten your learning curve while having fun and meeting new people.

You can also approach trying new recipes like planning a trip around the world through vegan food. This is something I still love doing today. Most traditional foods from cultures around the world are primarily plant-based, so this can be an enjoyable, educational, and ongoing experience. What your own traditional and cultural foods are will, of course, determine what's new to you, which could include Ethiopian, Indian, Mexican, Italian, Thai, Soul, Southern, and more. You'll find several recipes from these cuisines in this book.

STEP 9: PLAN YOUR MEALS

Planning your meals in advance can be an essential practice to help you gain confidence and relieve anxiety about what to eat each day. In the early stages of your vegan transition, you're more likely to rely on recipes from the Internet and cookbooks for meal ideas, as we talked about in step 8. But as you gain experience, you'll be more comfortable with pulling ingredients from the fridge and pantry to create meals without recipes.

Meal planning can also help you eat healthier because it can lead to cooking more meals at home, where you're in control of ingredients and portion sizes. Meal planning can also help you save money because you'll be more inclined to shop for what you planned for and less likely to buy on impulse.

To get started with planning your meals, you'll probably find it easiest to plan meals one week at a time. Keep in mind your schedule for the week and which days and evenings are extra busy so you can make quick and easy meals on those days or batch cook ahead of time on the weekends. For batch cooking, you can make a big pot of grains or soup on a Sunday, then freeze them in airtight containers for lunches and dinners during the week. You can also take one day to wash and dry greens, then store some in your salad spinner in the refrigerator so they're ready for salads, wraps, and sautés whenever you want them. And you can freeze some of the greens, in addition to freezing fruits like bananas and berries, so they're ready for morning smoothies.

Also, to keep your meal plan as simple as possible, choose meals with similar ingredients so you can make multiple dishes with them. For example, tempeh can be used for a veggie stir-fry on Monday and a panini on Wednesday. And black beans can be used for tacos on Tuesday and black bean soup on Thursday.

You can also streamline your meal plan by focusing on meals for dinner and just making extra for lunch the next day. That can save you time, energy, and stress around what to eat for lunch and dinner each day. For breakfast, you can keep it simple with a smoothie and overnight oats, breakfast pudding, or granola with nondairy milk.

Once you've done your meal plan for the week, create a grocery shopping list and consider keeping it on your phone. Then go out and get those ingredients! Most people tend to make one big grocery shopping trip on the weekend to one or more stores. If that's you, continue doing that as a new vegan. Just keep in mind that you may need to go to a new store or farmers' market that has more vegan ingredients.

One final tip, keep your weekly meal plan where it's visible, like the fridge, wall, or nook area in the kitchen. That way, you'll spark anticipation for all the healthy and delicious food you'll be enjoying during the week.

STEP 10: READ THE LABEL

As you transition to vegan foods, it's vital to know how to read food labels to spot hidden animal products in packaged foods that you might otherwise expect to be vegan. For example, some brands of veggie burgers contain dairy products. So if the label doesn't clearly state that the product is vegan, your best bet is to do a quick scan of the ingredients list. Here are five of the most common hidden animal ingredients to avoid.

NATURAL FLAVORS. These are additives that give a food product its flavor. In general, the Food and Drug Administration allows companies to hide ingredients under the term "natural flavors" as a way to protect their secret recipe. The concern here is that natural flavors could be animal-derived or plant-derived. Unless the product explicitly states that it's vegan, you have no way of knowing if the natural flavors are vegan, unless you ask the company directly.

WHEY. This is a watery substance derived from the fat and protein in milk during the cheese-making process. Whey is often found in foods that you might expect to be vegan, like certain brands of soy cheese and rice cheese. So read the ingredients list carefully or look for "vegan" on the label of nondairy cheeses. Whey can also be found in dry mixes, bakery products, ice cream, and other processed foods.

CASEIN. This is a milk protein that's also found in otherwise nondairy cheeses, as well as in ice cream, bakery products, cereals, breakfast bars, and granola.

CARMINE. This is a red dye in food products that comes from the bodies of dried female insects called cochineals. Carmine is found in juices and other drinks, fruit fillings, yogurt, ice cream, and other dairy products.

GELATIN. This is an animal protein from pigs or cows that's used as a thickening agent in foods like puddings, juice, frozen desserts, and the capsules used for vitamin supplements and pills.

For more information on hidden animal ingredients in vegan food products, check out the "Vegetarian Journal Guide to Food Ingredients" from the Vegetarian Resource Group, which can be found at VRG.org.

If this feels a bit overwhelming, keep in mind that the explosion of new vegan foods found on supermarket shelves around the country are usually labeled as vegan. But in cases where they aren't clearly labeled and you're unsure, just check the ingredients list. And even better, eat more foods that don't come in packages or that *do* have simple ingredients you easily recognize as fruits, vegetables, whole grains, beans, nuts, and seeds.

STEP 11: STAY ON BUDGET

The secret to eating vegan and healthy on the cheap is to get your staple ingredients from the bulk bins at the grocery store. This includes basics, such as whole grains, dried beans, nuts, seeds, and herbs and spices. It can also include common ingredients like dried fruits and vegetables, almond butter and other nut butters, sweeteners, and oils. Not only do you save money, but you also have control over the amount of food you purchase, so you can buy as little or as much as you need. And you won't be purchasing and later disposing of unnecessary food packaging.

On the other hand, the more processed and packaged vegan foods are, the more expensive they tend to be. For example, vegan versions of burgers, hot dogs, deli meats, chicken, cheese, and ice cream can cost as much or more than the animal versions.

Buying fresh, local food at farmers' markets and through community-supported agriculture (CSA) can also save you money. Of course, growing your own food, particularly fruits, vegetables, and herbs—whether in your backyard, balcony, windowsill, community garden, or elsewhere—can save you the most money, be healthier for you, and taste better.

When you do shop at the grocery store, it's best to buy fresh fruits and vegetables in season, when they're more abundant and prices tend to be lower as a result. Frozen fruit and vegetables can be affordable and healthy options as well, especially if they help you eat more produce throughout the year.

And what about spending money on organic fruits and vegetables? To help answer that question, check out the Environmental Working Group (EWG.org) for its free "Shopper's Guide to Pesticides in Produce." Each year, the EWG analyzes data from the US Department of Agriculture and the Food and Drug Administration on the amount of pesticide residue found in the nation's fresh produce supply. Based on this data, the guide ranks about fifty of the most popular fresh fruits and vegetables according to how much or how little pesticide residue they contain after being washed and, in some cases, peeled.

Most conventional produce is sprayed with pesticides, including fungicides, insecticides, and herbicides, and there are proven health risks associated with these toxic chemicals for farm workers and consumers. As a consumer, the EWG guide essentially lets you know which fruits and vegetables you can safely buy organic and nonorganic. That helps you stay healthy *and* save money.

And finally, remember that the money you spend on healthy food now can add years to your life and life to your years.

STEP 12: EAT OUT WITH EASE

It's easier than ever to keep your meals vegan and healthy when you eat out. Your first choice can be eating at vegan restaurants. There are more than six hundred all-vegan restaurants in the United States. In fact, there's at least one in every state. To find vegan (and vegetarian) restaurants in your area, check out HappyCow.net or VegDining.com or do an online search for local vegan restaurants.

Next, try what I refer to as world cuisine restaurants, where a large part of the menu is plant-based. It can be easy to find restaurants featuring cuisines from countries in Africa, Asia, North and South America, and Europe that are already vegan or can easily be made vegan.

More nonvegan restaurants are also offering vegan options to meet the ever-increasing demand. In fact, according to a 2016 Vegetarian Resource Group poll, more than one-third of the US population always or sometimes eats meatless meals when eating out. So when eating out, be sure to check out the online menu for vegan meals in advance. If you have any questions about how the dish is prepared, like whether the vegetables are sautéed in butter or oil, or whether any meat or dairy is used in the broth, sauce, or cream, just call the restaurant and ask.

If you can't check out the menu or call in advance, ask the waiters for their recommendations. You might be surprised to find there are unlabeled vegan options on the menu. Or the restaurant may have some vegan dishes not on the menu that they often make for vegan patrons who request them.

When you know your options, your choices for eating out as a vegan can be unlimited, so you can enjoy eating out just as much or more than you ever did.

STEP 13: KEEP A STASH

This is an aspect of going vegan that people don't often think about, but it's one that will help you maintain your new lifestyle in any situation. Keeping a stash means being prepared with your favorite healthy vegan snacks during those times when there's no other food available or when you're not sure if the food is vegan. Or when there is vegan food, but it's not as healthy as what you might normally eat. You'll encounter *many* situations like these, including receptions, meetings, concerts and shows, visits with family and friends, long commutes, waiting at the doctor's office or the DMV—you get the picture.

Whether the activity is planned or unexpected, keeping a stash will keep you prepared. It can also make your experience more enjoyable because you'll feel more relaxed, instead of worried about what you're going to eat. Even after thirty years as a vegan, I still keep a stash on hand, and it's a practice that's served me well over the years.

So what exactly should be in your stash? You want to keep it healthy, so that can include fruit, nuts, healthy food bars, air-popped popcorn, baked chips, whole-grain crackers, homemade whole-grain muffins, a PB&J sandwich on whole-grain bread, and much more. You want foods that don't need to be refrigerated or can be safely eaten within two hours of being taken out of the fridge. Check out "Snacks and Bites" in part 2 for more recipe ideas. And you'll want to keep your stash in your purse, bag, backpack, car, desk, refrigerator at work, or other convenient and accessible place.

Be sure to keep your stash replenished when you run low. You may also want to include a stash section on your grocery shopping list as a reminder to keep it stocked.

Keeping a stash can also help you save money and stay healthy because you're less likely to buy an overpriced, not-so-healthy snack on your way to or from an event or during an intermission. You're also less likely to overindulge once you do eat a full meal. So always keep a stash of your healthy favorites on hand and relax.

STEP 14: ENJOY THE JOURNEY

The last step is to enjoy your journey to becoming a vegan, with all of its joys and challenges. Once you begin, if you're inclined to want to rush through the transition process, try slowing down and being present. Experience it. Notice what it feels like. Notice what emotions come up for you. Journal about them. Exercise, meditate, laugh, reread the guidance in these fourteen steps, and lean on your support community to help you manage the inevitable stress that comes with changing the way you eat.

And if you slip up, be easy with yourself. Just start again the next day. Remember that as you go through the transition process, consistency is what matters. Every step you take makes a difference, every vegan meal counts. So take it one day at a time.

And also remember that with every vegan meal you eat, your taste buds will change for the better. Studies show that our taste buds physically change within just a few weeks of eating healthier foods. The more low-fat, low-sugar, and low-salt foods we eat, the better they taste. Our taste buds actually become more sensitive to and less wanting of higher doses of fat, salt, and sugar if we're reintroduced to them. So the longer you eat healthier, plant-based foods, the more you'll want to eat them.

And once you fully transition from an omnivore to a vegan, the next phase of your journey begins—that of actually being vegan. And as time passes, you'll find that being vegan gets easier and easier, to the point that it becomes your new normal. It becomes effortless and second nature. And you'll come to know that being vegan is a path, not a destination. It's part of the foundation of a healthy life that allows you to pursue your purpose and passions with greater ease and joy.

So celebrate yourself. Revel in your decision to go vegan. You are making one of the most life-changing and life-affirming decisions you can ever make. You'll look back at yourself years from now with deep gratitude and you'll be your own source of inspiration.

3

Creating a Vegan Kitchen

When you start eating healthier, your food preparation becomes much easier when you already have your kitchen set up with the tools you need. And stocking your pantry with colorful vegan ingredients will help get your creative juices flowing. Here are some ideas to get you started.

KITCHEN TOOLS AND TIPS

These are the time-saving tools that we use most in our kitchens, along with tips on how to use them. You may already have many of these, which should give you a jumpstart to cooking more vegan food right away.

CHEF'S KNIFE AND PARING KNIFE

Apart from your own hands, these are probably your most essential tools in the kitchen. If you cook from scratch most of the time (which I hope you do), then you'll be doing a lot of vegetable chopping, which requires good knives. Be sure to get a chef's knife with a size and weight that fits well in your hand. And don't forget the knife sharpener. Keeping your knives sharp will help make chopping much easier and will protect your hands from slips that happen more readily with a dull knife.

CITRUS JUICER

I use my citrus juicer just about every day for freshly squeezed lemon juice. I find it's much easier to extract more juice this way than by hand.

ELECTRIC CROCK-POT

Using an electric Crock-Pot (or slow cooker) makes it easy to cook a big batch of beans, rice, stew, chili, and other dishes on the weekend to eat from during the week. Or you can use it to cook while you're away from home or sleeping or just doing other things. You won't have to constantly check on the food, and when it's hot outside, you won't have to turn on the stove or oven. Crock-Pots are also energy efficient, which makes them cost-effective to use, as well.

FOOD PROCESSOR

Chopping vegetables, onions, garlic, and nuts are much easier with a food processor. It's also great for easily making sauces, dips, and pesto.

GLASS CANNING JARS

These are my favorite containers for storing my leftover smoothies and green drinks in the refrigerator and they are great portable containers. I also use them to store dry staples like beans, nuts, seeds, and whole grains.

HIGH-SPEED BLENDER

I highly recommend investing in a good-quality high-speed blender if you can, because it makes eating more plant foods a breeze. I use a Vitamix, which can be a bit costly, but it lasts. I've used mine every day for many years to make daily green smoothies or vegetable drinks that come out silky smooth, with no or low visible pulp. I also use it to blend just about anything else, from soups to pie fillings to cashew cream to puréed fruit.

IMMERSION BLENDER

A handheld immersion blender is a convenient, lightweight, and simple way to blend and mix ingredients directly in a bowl or hot soup pot, eliminating the extra steps needed to place ingredients in a standard mixer or blender. And they're surprisingly affordable, which makes them even more appealing.

KITCHEN SCISSORS

I use my kitchen scissors to cut my baked tortillas and pitas into chip-size pieces for dips and soups. They also work well to cut stalks away from greens, especially if neatness counts for making wraps or rolls.

SALAD SPINNER

Besides my blender, this is probably my most-used kitchen tool. Salad spinners help take away the pain of washing and drying dark leafy greens. You can easily wash and spin-dry your greens without the mess, then store them in the refrigerator right in the spinner. Here's my secret: I actually have two salad spinners. One I use to store my washed and cleaned kale for my daily salads. And the other I use to wash, dry, and store the other vegetables I eat during the week, including broccoli, collards, mustard greens, chard, and others.

SPIRAL SLICER

A spiral slicer (or spiralizer) is especially useful to help you eat more fresh vegetables during the summer months when there's much more fresh produce available. You can use the spiral slicer to make paper-thin slices of a variety of vegetables or spaghetti-like strands of zucchini and squash. You can also use it to julienne strips and half rounds of vegetables to easily add to salads, stir-fries, and soups or to dip in hummus or salsa. You can take many dishes from plain to gorgeous with this tool.

STAINLESS STEEL TONGS

In addition to using stainless steel tongs to toss salads, I use them to toss leafy greens, string beans, or bell peppers when I'm lightly sautéing them on the stove. I also use them to turn grilled tempeh or tofu in the oven. Be sure to get long tongs to handle these hot cooking tasks.

WHISK

Stainless steel whisks are essential for stirring dry mixes when baking or when mixing together marinades. You can also use them to stir ingredients directly into a soup pot on the stove.

When you're using these kitchen tools, be sure to have designated counter space that's cleared for food preparation. And be sure the appliances you use the most are easily accessible so you're more likely to use them.

STOCKING THE VEGAN PANTRY

Having a well-stocked kitchen is a great way to have everything at your fingertips to prepare healthy, well-balanced meals each day. Here's a list of vegan pantry staples that we keep on hand in our kitchens. Many of these staples are used in the recipes in this book, as well. If some of these foods are new to you, don't worry—I provide descriptions of less-familiar items. This list is a general resource, so don't feel you need to stock all of these foods in your kitchen. You can use it as a guide to create your own master list to help you get started or continue on your vegan journey with confidence.

FRUITS AND VEGETABLES

It's always a good idea to keep a bowl of colorful fresh fruits and vegetables on your kitchen counter or someplace visible in your refrigerator where you can easily be reminded to eat them. When choosing fruits and vegetables, go for your favorites, but also focus on color and variety. The different colors of fruits and vegetables (as well as whole grains, beans, nuts, and seeds) reflect their distinct antioxidant content, so strive to eat from the rainbow each week to get their full benefits. Remember, Health Is in the Hue. Here are some examples.

FOR RED FRUITS AND VEGGIES, the major antioxidant that provides their pigment is lycopene, which is known to help reduce the risk of heart attack and prostate cancer. Red fruits and vegetables that you'll want to eat a variety of include:

RED FRUITS	RED VEGETABLES
Apples	Beets
Cherries	Radishes
Cranberries	Red bell peppers
Grapefruit	(which are technically a fruit)
Pears	Red onions
Pomegranates	
Raspberries	
Strawberries	
Tomatoes	
Watermelon	

YELLOW AND ORANGE FRUITS AND VEGETABLES are known for their high beta-carotene content, which converts to vitamin A in the body and helps to not only improve vision and reduce the risk of cataracts, but prevent stomach, lung, and esophagus cancers, as well. Yellow and orange fruits and vegetables include:

YELLOW AND ORANGE FRUITS	YELLOW AND ORANGE VEGETABLES
Apricots	Carrots
Cantaloupe	Orange and yellow peppers
Lemons	Pumpkins
Mangos	Squash
Oranges	Sweet potatoes
Peaches	Yellow corn
Pineapples	
Yellow apples	
Yellow pears	

BLUE AND PURPLE FRUITS AND VEGETABLES are rich in brain-boosting anthocyanidins (as mentioned in chapter 2), along with other health-promoting antioxidants. These fruits and vegetables include:

BLUE AND PURPLE FRUITS	BLUE AND PURPLE VEGETABLES
Black currants	Blue or purple potatoes
Blackberries	Eggplants
Blueberries	Purple bell peppers
Plums	Purple cabbage
Prunes	
Purple figs	
Purple grapes	
Raisins	

BROWN, TAN, CREAM, AND WHITE FRUITS AND VEGETABLES include garlic and onions, which contain the phytonutrient allicin, a type of anti-viral compound that helps ward off infections, and lowers blood pressure and cholesterol. Fruits and vegetables in this color group include:

BROWN, TAN, CREAM, AND WHITE FRUITS
Bananas
Brown pears
Dates
White peaches

BROWN, TAN, CREAM, AND WHITE VEGETABLES
Cauliflower
Garlic
Ginger
Mushrooms
Onions
Shallots
Turnips
White corn

AND LASTLY, THERE ARE GREEN FRUITS AND VEGETABLES, which we all know are healthy. I've previously mentioned two antioxidants found in these foods: lutein, which promotes eye health and decreases the risk of macular degeneration, and vitamin K, which helps build strong bones. Green fruits and vegetables include:

GREEN FRUITS
Avocados
Green apples
Green grapes
Honeydew
Kiwis
Limes

GREEN VEGETABLES
Arugula
Bok choy
Broccoli
Brussels sprouts
Celery
Chard
Collards
Cucumbers
  (which are technically a fruit)
Dandelion greens
Green beans
Green cabbage
Kale
Mustard greens
Parsley
Spinach
Zucchini

BEANS

Beans pack the biggest protein punch of all plant-based foods. They're also high in fiber, iron, magnesium, potassium, and folate, collectively. Super nutritious, beans have been shown to dramatically decrease cholesterol levels, reduce the risk of heart disease, and increase longevity. They're also versatile and inexpensive. As with fruits and vegetables, you want to eat beans in a variety of colors to get their full range of antioxidant benefits. Getting dried beans from the bulk bin is the most economical. But for convenience, cooked beans from a carton or a BPA-free can are fine, as long as the ingredients are just beans and water, with no added salt or preservatives. (BPA or bisphenol A is a harmful chemical found in the lining of food cans, so look for "BPA-free" or "Non-BPA Lining" on the label.)

SOME OF OUR FAVORITES ARE:

Black beans

Black-eyed peas

Butter beans

Cannellini

Chickpeas (garbanzos)

Lentils

Lima beans

Pinto beans

Red kidney beans

Split peas

You can also eat beans as burgers, soup, dip, tempeh, or tofu. If you're new to these latter two, read on.

TEMPEH. Tempeh is made by fermenting whole soybeans into a chewy, firm, and dense patty. Because it's made from whole soybeans, it's more nutritious than tofu. Tempeh doesn't have much flavor on its own, but it comes to life when sliced and marinated in your favorite sauce before stir-frying, oven-baking, or grilling.

TOFU. Tofu is made by coagulating curdled soy milk into a soft or firm block. Like tempeh, tofu soaks up the flavor of whatever sauces and seasonings are used to prepare it. Soft tofu is typically used for dips, puddings, and baked desserts, while firm tofu is used for stir-frying, oven-baking, or grilling.

Be sure to use organic tempeh or tofu to avoid otherwise genetically modified or pesticide-sprayed soy products.

NUTS AND SEEDS

High in protein, healthy fats, fiber, calcium, and other important vitamins and minerals, nuts and seeds are a key part of a healthy vegan diet. Studies show that eating a handful of nuts every day cuts your risk of having a heart attack in half, whereas *not* eating nuts every day doubles your risk of dying from heart disease.

OUR FAVORITE NUTS INCLUDE:

Almonds

Cashews

Macadamias

Pecans

Pine nuts

Pistachios

Pumpkin seeds

Sunflower seeds

Walnuts

SEEDS:

Chia seeds

Flax seeds

Hemp seeds

In our daily green smoothies, we usually add seeds, which are high in fiber and essential omega-3 fatty acids needed for proper cell functioning.

NUT AND SEED BUTTERS

If you like nut and seed butters for their taste, you'll love them for their health benefits, too. Eating a tablespoon of nut butter a day (or a handful of nuts) has been found to significantly reduce the chance that diabetic women will have a heart attack. Choose from raw nut butters like almond, cashew, and tahini (made from sesame seeds). Or better yet, make your own and save money because store-bought versions, particularly raw almond butter, can be pricey.

WHOLE GRAINS

What's the difference between whole grains and refined or processed grains? Whole grains have their healthy fiber, bran, vitamins, minerals, and phytonutrients intact.

SOME EXAMPLES OF WHOLE GRAINS ARE:

Barley	Millet
Bulgur	Oats
Corn	Rice (black, brown, and wild)

There's also quinoa (KEEN-wah), which is actually a seed but eaten like a grain. Quinoa is prized for its high protein content and easy digestibility. It's also high in fiber, iron, and vitamin E. Quinoa comes in black, red, and tan varieties, with tan being the most commonly used.

WHOLE-GRAIN FLOURS FOR BAKING

THE MOST COMMON WHOLE-GRAIN FLOURS USED FOR BAKING INCLUDE:

Cornmeal	Whole wheat flour
Oat flour	Whole wheat pastry flour
Whole spelt flour	

Less commonly known is white whole wheat flour, which is a 100 percent whole-grain flour made from hard white wheat berries instead of the hard red wheat berries used for whole wheat flour. It can be used instead of whole wheat flour in baking for a lighter color and milder taste.

COMMON GLUTEN-FREE WHOLE-GRAIN FLOURS INCLUDE:

Almond flour	Quinoa flour
Brown rice flour	Teff flour
Coconut flour	

Below are some additional ingredients we use in baking that may be new to you:

ALMOND MEAL. This is coarsely ground blanched almonds with the skin intact that we use in a few of the pie crusts and thicker salad dressings in the recipes in this book. Almond meal has a heavier texture than almond flour, which is finely ground blanched almonds with the skin removed and is often used as a gluten-free flour for airy cakes.

ARROWROOT. This is a fine, starchy powder derived from the arrowroot plant. It's most often used as a thickener for pies, sauces, and soups.

OAT BRAN. High in fiber and B vitamins, oat bran is used to add nutritional punch to foods and to increase the oat flavor.

WHOLE-GRAIN PASTAS AND NOODLES

If you're a noodle lover, it's a good idea to keep an ample supply of different sizes and shapes of whole-grain pastas in your pantry.

SOME USEFUL SHAPES TO HAVE ON HAND INCLUDE:

Angel hair	Rotini (or spirals)
Fettuccine	Spaghetti
Linguini	Ziti
Penne	

ASIAN NOODLES VARIETIES, INCLUDING:

Bean thread noodles	Soba
Rice noodles	Udon

These varieties of whole-grain pastas and noodles are available in health food stores and well-stocked supermarkets.

HERBS AND SPICES

For the best flavor and antioxidant power, make fresh herbs and spices your first choice—either those that you grow yourself, get at a farmers' market, or pick up from a grocery store. Keep them in a jar of water on your kitchen counter for just a couple of days or as packaged in the fridge.

THE BASICS INCLUDE:

Basil

Cilantro

Oregano

Parsley

Rosemary

Thyme

FOR DRIED HERBS, KEEP A GOOD RANGE OF COMMONLY USED VARIETIES ON HAND, ESPECIALLY:

All-purpose, salt-free, herb-and-spice blend

Good-quality curry powder

Italian herb seasoning blend

Hot peppers (dried)

Mushrooms (dried)

Seaweeds (dried or toasted nori sheets and dulse and kelp granules. These are available at health food stores and Asian food markets).

Nutritional yeast is also essential to keep stocked in your pantry. This vegan favorite is a type of yeast grown on molasses that is heated (to deactivate the yeast), harvested, washed, and packaged as flakes or powder. You can use it wherever you would add parmesan cheese or salt. Depending on the brand, it can be a great source of B vitamins and many other nutrients.

PREPARED CONDIMENTS AND SAUCES

Basics include the following (be sure to look for low-sodium and sugar-free varieties as your first choice):

Apple cider vinegar

Balsamic vinegar

BBQ sauce

Black bean stir-fry sauce

Hoisin sauce

Marinara

Mustard

Peanut sauce

Pesto

Salsa

Vegan mayo

Below are some additional condiments we use in the recipes that may be new to you.

COCONUT AMINOS. This sauce is made from coconut tree sap and has a slightly sweet and salty flavor. It's often used instead of soy sauce or tamari (see below) because it's gluten-free and soy-free and has a lower sodium content.

COCONUT MILK. Depending on the recipe, we use either light (low-fat) or regular (full fat) canned coconut milk from "BPA-free" or "Non-BPA lined" cans, just as we do with canned beans (see page 52).

COCONUT VINEGAR. Fermented from the sap of coconut blossoms, nutrient-rich coconut vinegar can be used instead of apple cider vinegar.

MISO. A Japanese condiment made from fermented soybeans or other beans combined with whole grains (like barley or brown rice), sea salt, and cultures to form a thick paste commonly used to season soups and sauces.

TAMARI. A type of Japanese soy sauce made from fermented soybeans that does not contain wheat and tastes less salty than more commonly used soy sauces.

Sweeteners

THERE ARE FIVE TYPES OF SWEETENERS USED IN THE RECIPES IN THIS BOOK:

Fruits

Maple syrup

Molasses

Date sugar: Made from dried and ground dates, date sugar is a healthier whole-food sweetener that's high in fiber, potassium, and iron. It can replace white table sugar one-to-one.

Coconut sugar: Made from the dried sap of the coconut palm tree flower, coconut sugar contains calcium, iron, zinc, and potassium. It can also replace white table sugar one-to-one.

Oils

Many whole plant-based foods come with naturally occurring healthy fats or oils, including nuts, seeds, olives, avocados, and whole grains. So it's not necessary to have added oils in your diet. That said, you can use oils in small amounts for added flavor, as we do in the recipes. You can sauté or stir-fry for 5–10 minutes on a low or medium flame. Additionally, you can use these as either poured oils on foods like salads or as ingredients in baking.

BASIC OILS

Extra-virgin olive oil ("extra-virgin" means it comes from the first press of the fruit and retains much of its nutrient content)

Extra-virgin coconut oil

Grapeseed oil

Safflower oil

Sesame oil

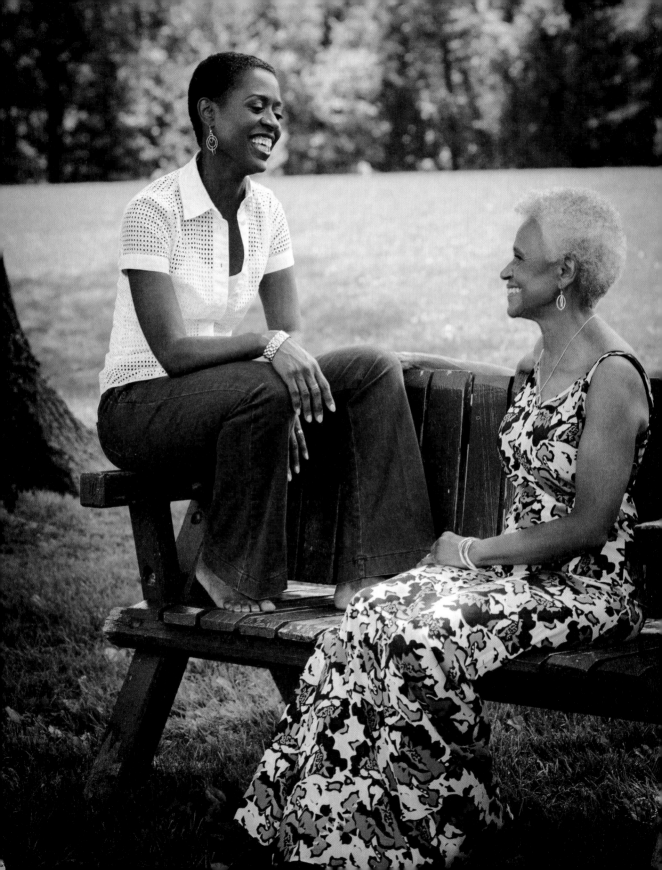

part two

100 Delicious Recipes
for a Long
and Healthy Life

Look for these phrases at the bottom of recipes that incorporate superfoods for greater health and longevity, and that reflect some of our Fab Five Food Rules:

AGELESS ANTIOXIDANTS Features superfoods that prevent premature aging

BRAIN BOOSTER Features superfoods that promote healthy brain functioning

HEALTH IS IN THE HUE Features ingredients with a variety of health-promoting colors

LONGEVITY LOVER Features superfoods that decrease the risk of chronic diseases and premature death

PROTEIN DREAM Features ingredients high in protein

SMOOTH SKIN Features superfoods that help skin stay smooth and reduce wrinkles

STRONG BONES Features superfoods that strengthen bones and muscles

SUPER GREENS Features superfood dark leafy greens, the most nutritious of all foods

VISION MISSION Features superfoods that improve vision

4

Smoothies & Drinks

In this chapter, you'll find recipes for Tracye's Daily Green Smoothie and Mary's Daily Green Smoothie, the nutrient-rich green drinks we have each day. They're an essential part of our daily dose of dark leafy greens—one of the main ingredients for our radiant health. The refreshing drinks you'll also find here include some of our favorites, like Sparkling Basil Limonade and Mango Lassi Smoothie. And some healthy indulgences, like Cashew Nog and Hot Chocolate with Coconut Cream and Cacao Nibs.

Tracye's Daily Green Smoothie

Mary's Daily Green Smoothie

Pineapple Spinach Smoothie

Mango Lassi Smoothie

Sweet Potato Smoothie

Watermelon Kiwi Lime Smoothie

Berry Beet Smoothie

Sparkling Basil Limonade

Green Tea with Ginger and Cardamom

Liquid Sunshine Dandelion Lemon Drink

the Concoction

Cashew Nog

Hot Chocolate with Coconut Cream and Cacao Nibs

Vanilla Almond Milk

Coconut Cashew Milk

Daily Green Smoothie

I drink a green smoothie almost every day. It usually includes dandelion greens, but I also switch it up for more nutrient variety with kale, spinach, or collards. As the most nutritious of all foods, dark leafy greens protect against heart disease, cancer, and stroke—our top killers—and premature aging of the brain, eyes, bones, and skin.

12 leaves dandelion greens

1 banana, or 1 avocado, pitted

1 cup fresh or frozen berries (blueberries, blackberries, strawberries, or raspberries)

1-inch piece ginger, peeled

3 tablespoons ground hemp seeds

Place all ingredients and 3 cups water in a high-speed blender and blend until smooth. Serve immediately.

MAKES 3-4 SERVINGS

MARY'S
DAILY GREEN SMOOTHIE

My mom drinks about 2 to 3 cups of green smoothie every day. She has the first cup before her morning exercise classes because the protein from the flax or hemp seeds, along with the complex carbohydrates from all the ingredients, help sustain her energy level. She drinks the rest throughout the day. She uses different combinations of green leafy vegetables and fruits on a regular basis to be sure she's getting the health benefits of a variety of nutrients throughout the week.

Place all ingredients and 3 cups water in a high-speed blender and blend until smooth. Serve immediately.

MAKES 3-4 SERVINGS

4–5 leaves kale, bottom stems removed

1-inch piece ginger, peeled

1 medium apple, cored and halved

½ cup blueberries

1 teaspoon freshly squeezed lemon juice (about ¼ lemon)

2 tablespoons flax seeds

3 tablespoons ground hemp seeds (optional)

AGELESS ANTIOXIDANTS   BRAIN BOOSTER   HEALTH IS IN THE HUE   LONGEVITY LOVER
PROTEIN DREAM   SMOOTH SKIN   STRONG BONES   SUPER GREENS   VISION MISSION

63

PINEAPPLE SPINACH SMOOTHIE

In addition to being rich in iron, spinach is high in ageless antioxidants that promote long-term vision health and help prevent cataracts and macular degeneration. This smoothie blends spinach with sweet pineapple and creamy avocado, which adds healthy fats and helps you feel full longer.

2 cups frozen pineapple chunks
½ avocado, pitted
2 cups fresh or frozen spinach

In a blender, combine all the ingredients with 1¼ cups water. Blend until smooth. Serve immediately.

MAKES 2 SERVINGS

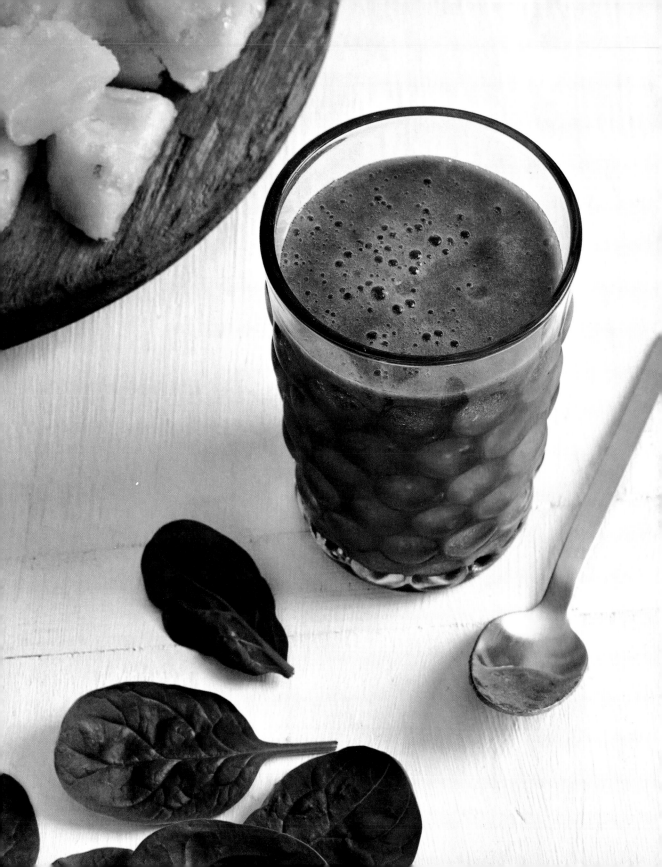

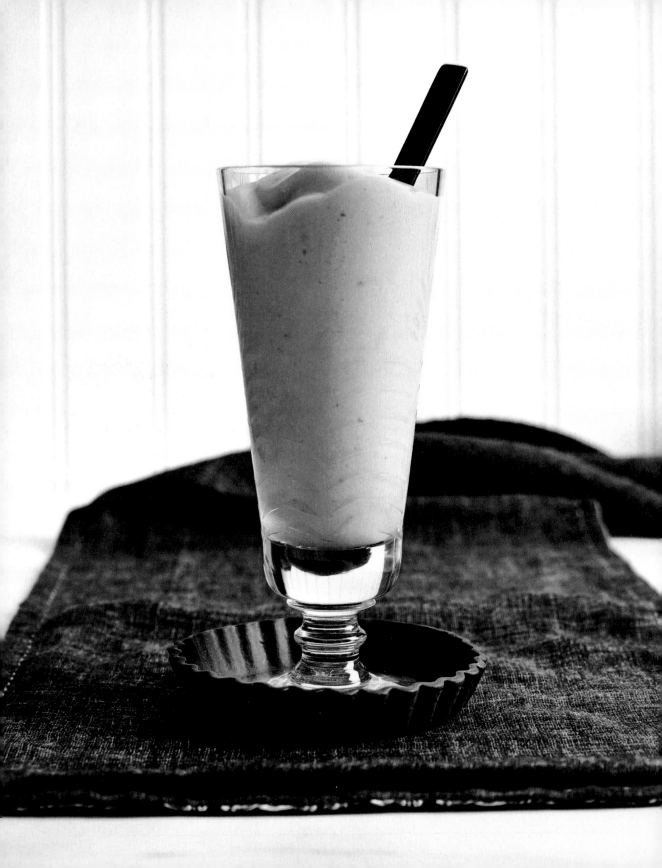

MANGO LASSI SMOOTHIE

This is a vegan twist on the traditional Indian lassi made with yogurt. It combines three of my favorite fruits, mango, coconut, and dates, with one of my favorite spices, cardamom—a good source of colon-cleansing fiber, bone-protecting manganese, and cancer-fighting compounds. This drink is pure bliss. I think you'll agree!

In a blender, combine all ingredients. Blend until smooth. For a thinner drink, add 1 additional tablespoon at a time of coconut milk or water. Serve immediately.

MAKES 2 SERVINGS

1 cup coconut milk
(light or regular)

2 cups frozen mango chunks

½ banana

½ teaspoon freshly squeezed lemon
juice (about ⅛ lemon)

1 Medjool date, pitted
Pinch sea salt

¼ teaspoon ground cardamom

Sweet Potato Smoothie

I whipped up this smoothie when I wanted to create something interesting and healthy for dessert with what I had on hand. I grabbed what was left in the fruit bowl and voilà! It turned out to be one of my best smoothies ever. Not only because it's delicious, but because sweet potatoes are so nutritious. Their ageless antioxidants include beta carotene, which helps reduce the risk for cancer, and vitamin A, which decreases the risk for vision deterioration as we get older.

3 cups Vanilla Almond Milk (page 80)

½ frozen banana

1 medium sweet potato, roasted, peeled, and mashed

1 tablespoon chopped walnuts

In a blender, add almond milk, banana, and sweet potato. Blend until smooth and creamy. To serve, pour into glasses and sprinkle chopped walnuts on top.

MAKES 3-4 SERVINGS

WATERMELON KIWI LIME SMOOTHIE

The sweet, citrusy, and tart combination of this smoothie makes it a perfect cold summertime drink. To make this drink a nutritional powerhouse, without taking away from its refreshing flavor, try adding a cup of frozen spinach. It's another great way to get your daily dose of health- and longevity-promoting dark leafy greens.

Place all the ingredients in a blender and blend until smooth. Chill and serve over ice.

MAKES 2-3 SERVINGS

2 cups watermelon chunks, cut small (should make about 2 cups of juice)

1 tablespoon freshly squeezed lime juice (about ½ medium lime)

1 small kiwi, peeled

BERRY BEET SMOOTHIE

This smoothie is as delicious as it is nutritious. The berries are rich in ageless antioxidants that help improve brain function as we get older and the beets are high in iron, vitamin C, and potassium, among other essential nutrients. The deep crimson color reflects the presence of these health-promoting compounds, and it's a perfect example of what we mean by the Health Is in the Hue.

½ medium beet, peeled and roughly chopped

½ cup frozen strawberries

½ cup frozen raspberries

1 medium orange, peeled and seeded

1 Medjool date, pitted

½ cup unsweetened almond milk

¼ teaspoon peeled and grated ginger

Place all the ingredients in a blender and blend until smooth. Serve immediately.

MAKES 2 SERVINGS

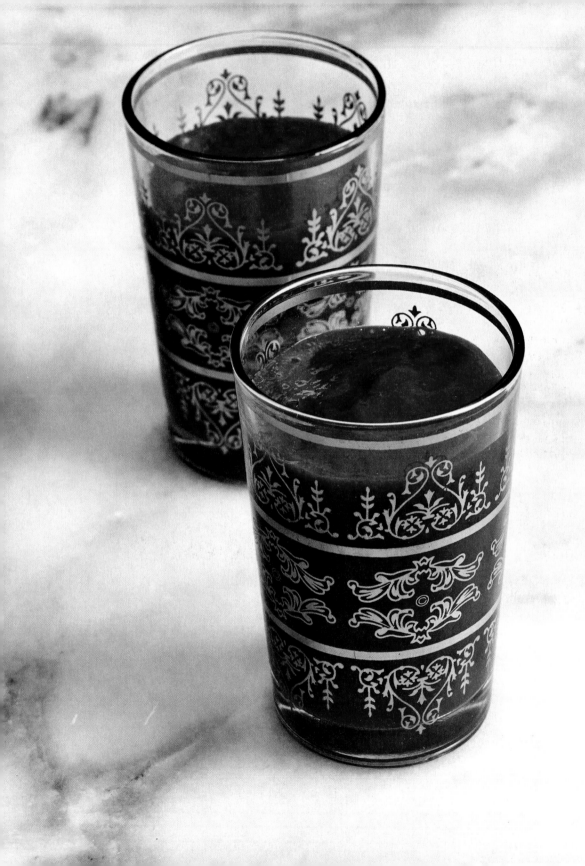

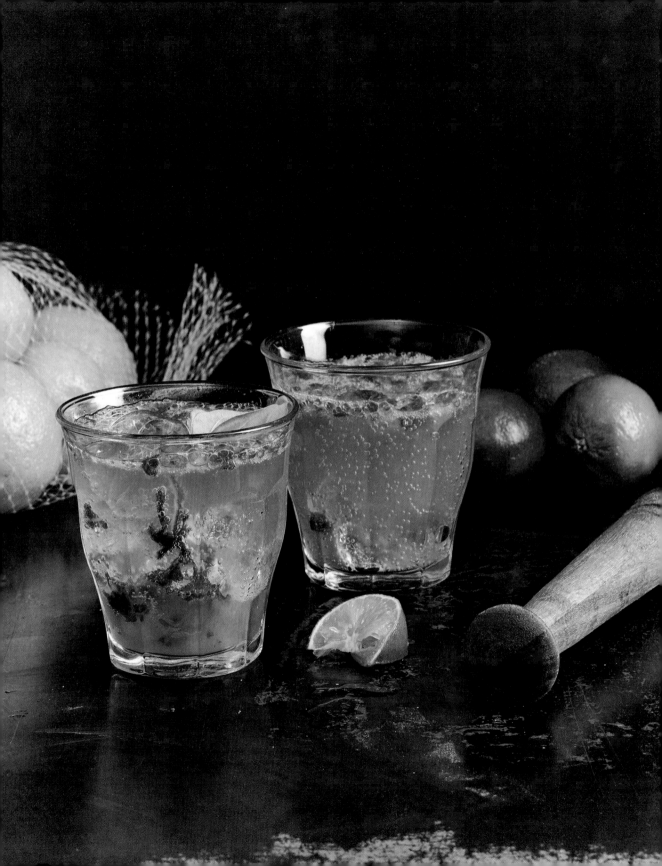

Sparkling Basil Limonade

This light, refreshing drink was inspired by the only soda we ever had in the house growing up: ginger ale. I think it sparked my lifelong love of sparkling water.

In a small pitcher, combine the basil, lime juice, lemon juice, and sugar. Use a wooden spoon to press down on and slightly bruise the leaves so more of the flavor will be incorporated into the drink. Add the sparkling water and ice cubes. Stir and serve immediately.

MAKES 2 SERVINGS

8 large basil leaves

2 tablespoons freshly squeezed lime juice (about 1 medium lime)

2 tablespoons freshly squeezed lemon juice (about 1 medium lemon)

1 teaspoon coconut sugar (or more, to taste)

3 cups sparkling water

1 cup ice cubes

GREEN TEA
with GINGER AND CARDAMOM

The antioxidant power of green tea makes it one of the healthiest drinks you can consume. It's been shown to decrease the risk for heart disease, stroke, and certain cancers (including breast, prostate, and colon cancers), and increase longevity. This recipe combines green tea with ginger and cancer-fighting cardamom for even more antioxidant benefits.

2 tablespoons peeled and roughly chopped ginger

4 whole cardamom pods, roughly chopped

1 green tea bag or 1 teaspoon loose green tea

½ teaspoon coconut sugar or more, to taste (optional)

In a large pot, add 3 cups water, ginger, and cardamom and bring to a boil. Reduce the heat to low and simmer for 10 minutes. Add the green tea to the ginger mixture and let brew until it reaches your desired strength. Strain with a tea strainer, if using loose tea. Stir in coconut sugar. Serve hot.

MAKES 2 SERVINGS

Dandelion Lemon Drink

This drink is the true secret to my glow! I drink about 2 cups almost every day. Dandelion greens are nutrient powerhouses, especially high in skin-nurturing vitamin A, vision-protecting lutein, bone-strengthening vitamin K, and colon-cleansing fiber. And of all the dark leafy greens I eat, dandelions just do something extra for me. When I drink it in the morning, it completely calms my mood and makes me feel balanced and clear as I start my day. I call it my liquid sunshine. Dandelion greens are typically available at health-food stores.

Place dandelion greens, lemon juice, and 2 cups water in a high-speed blender. Blend on highest speed until the greens turn to liquid, 5 to 10 seconds. For a cold drink, add in 3 to 4 ice cubes and blend for another few seconds. Serve immediately.

1   bunch dandelion greens
    (about 30 to 40 small leaves or
    10 to 20 large leaves)
⅓   cup freshly squeezed lemon juice
    (about 1 large lemon)

MAKES 2-3 SERVINGS

the
CONCOCTION

Family reunions, birthdays, the holidays—these are all special times that can mean feasting on more celebration foods than usual. And all that indulging can create excess mucus and congestion in our bodies. So when you feel a cold coming on, try this drink to knock it right out. My mother first whipped it up a few years ago, and trust me, it works! But be warned, you *will* smell like garlic. Chomp on a few sprigs of fresh parsley to cut the aroma and your peeps will thank you.

3–4 large garlic cloves
 1 small red onion, quartered
 1 large tomato
 1 large lemon, unpeeled, quartered
 ½ teaspoon cayenne (depending on
     your tolerance for heat)
4–5 sprigs parsley

Place all the ingredients, except parsley, in a high-speed blender and blend until smooth. No water needed. Drink immediately. Repeat as necessary. Chew on the parsley as a breath freshener.

MAKES 2 SERVINGS

CASHEW NOG

Inspired by the eggnog I loved as a child, this grown-up version is tastier, healthier, and more refreshing than the dairy version. It's spiced with antioxidant-rich cinnamon and cloves, which protect against damaging free radicals that can lead to premature aging. For an equally flavorful twist, try swapping the cloves for cardamom.

Place all ingredients in a blender with 3 cups water and blend until smooth and creamy. Chill and serve.

MAKES 3-4 SERVINGS

1½ cups raw cashews, soaked in water for 1 hour and drained

4 Medjool dates, pitted

1 teaspoon vanilla extract

¼ teaspoon cinnamon

⅛ teaspoon cloves

HOT CHOCOLATE
with COCONUT CREAM AND CACAO NIBS

There's nothing like sipping a cup of hot chocolate on a cold winter's day. But if you're like me, you can really drink it all year round. Protein-rich cashew milk and cashew cream are what give this hot chocolate its rich, indulgent flavor.

1   cup Coconut Cashew Milk
    (page 81)

2   tablespoons unsweetened
    cocoa powder

2   tablespoons coconut cream
    (thick part only; save liquid for
    other uses)

¼   teaspoon cacao nibs

In a blender, combine milk and cocoa powder and blend until smooth, about 1 minute. Put mixture in a pot and simmer on low heat until hot, about 5 minutes. Once hot, pour into mugs and garnish with the thick coconut cream and cacao nibs. Serve hot.

MAKES 2 SERVINGS

What's Coconut Cream?

Coconut cream is the thick, rich, paste-like cream that rises to the top of a can of coconut milk. Coconut cream is most often used to replace whipped cream. You can buy a can of coconut cream (in store or online) or a can of coconut milk. If you buy canned coconut milk and the cream is not already formed on top, you'll need to refrigerate the can for about 24 to 48 hours for the coconut cream to solidify, separate, and rise to the top. Also, keep in mind that coconut cream is not the same as cream of coconut, which is a presweetened coconut cream often used in drinks like Piña Colada.

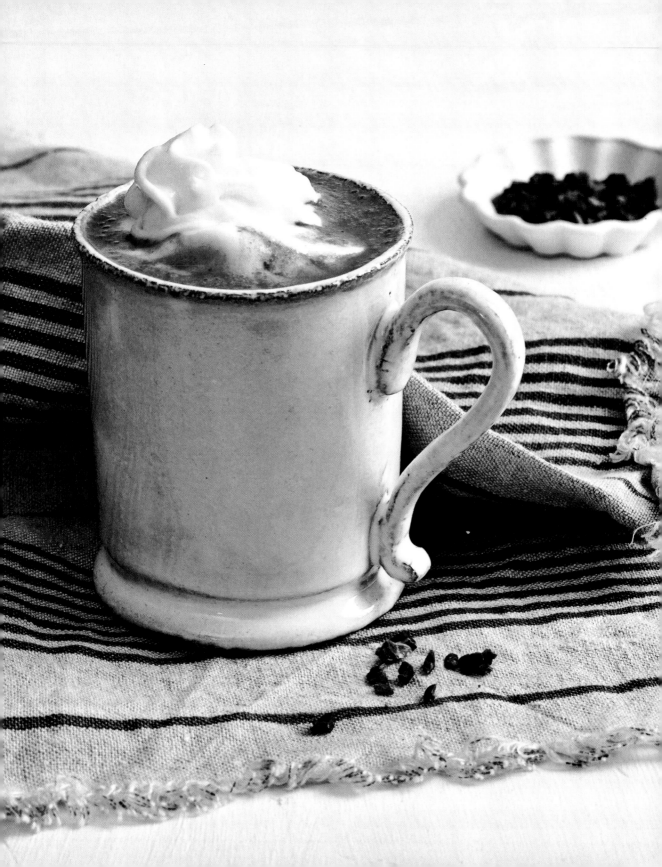

Vanilla Almond Milk

While store-bought almond milk is convenient, it's healthier and cheaper to make your own. This protein- and calcium-rich recipe calls for just three simple ingredients with water, so it's easy to DIY in no time.

1 cup raw almonds, soaked overnight and drained

1 vanilla bean, cut in half lengthwise and seeded, or ¼ teaspoon vanilla extract

3 Medjool dates, pitted

Place almonds in a blender with 3 cups water and blend until smooth, about 1 minute. Strain almond milk through a fine sieve or cheesecloth. Pour the almond milk back in the blender and add the vanilla and dates. Blend until the dates are completely incorporated, about 1 minute. Chill and serve. The almond milk will last 2 to 3 days in the fridge.

TIPS To make chocolate milk, blend in 3 teaspoons cocoa powder.

To make the almond milk sweeter, add 1 to 2 more dates, to taste. For less sweet milk, you can skip the dates altogether or add in one date at a time, tasting as you go.

MAKES 3-4 SERVINGS

COCONUT CASHEW MILK

Packed with protein, this drink is great on its own or paired with Vanilla Cinnamon Granola with Almonds (page 94) or Apple Raisin Granola with Pumpkin Seeds (page 96).

Place all ingredients in a blender and blend on the highest speed. For thinner nut milk, strain the liquid through a fine sieve or cheesecloth. Chill and serve.

MAKES 4 SERVINGS

1½ cups raw cashews, soaked in water for 1 hour and drained

3 cups coconut water

3 Medjool dates, pitted

½ teaspoon vanilla extract

AGELESS ANTIOXIDANTS   BRAIN BOOSTER   HEALTH IS IN THE HUB   LONGEVITY LOVER
PROTEIN DREAM   SMOOTH SKIN   STRONG BONES   SUPER GREENS   VISION MISSION

81

5

Breakfast

Several of the recipes in this section are perfect for busy weekday mornings. You can make Blueberry Muffins and Banana Walnut Muffins in batches over the weekend to grab and go during the week. And you can prep Overnight Oats with Pear and Pistachios and Chia Berry Breakfast Pudding the night before. Other recipes, like Maple French Toast with Strawberries and Curried Tofu Scramble with Shiitake Mushrooms, are best savored over leisurely Sunday brunches with family and friends.

Avocado Toast

Sunrise Smoothie Bowl

Chia Berry Breakfast Pudding

Overnight Oats with Pear and Pistachios

Banana Walnut Muffins

Blueberry Muffins

Vanilla Cinnamon Granola with Almonds

Apple Raisin Granola with Pumpkin Seeds

Home Fries

Maple French Toast with Strawberries

Home-Style Grits

Curried Tofu Scramble with Shiitake Mushrooms

Avocado Quesadillas with Salsa and Cashew Sour Cream

AVOCADO TOAST

Avocados are high in vision-protecting lutein, muscle-strengthening potassium, and colon-cleansing fiber. They're also an excellent source of healthy monounsaturated fat, which lowers harmful LDL cholesterol and decreases the risk of heart disease. This avocado toast recipe feels like an indulgence—and it's good for you!

4 (½-inch-thick) slices whole-grain bread

1 tablespoon extra-virgin olive oil

2 medium avocados, pitted and mashed

1 tablespoon rice vinegar

¼ teaspoon sea salt

½ red onion, thinly sliced

1 tablespoon sesame seeds (black, brown, or mixed)

1 teaspoon finely chopped chives

1 teaspoon chili flakes

1 lemon wedge (optional)

2 edible flowers, such as blue coral flower petals (optional)

Preheat oven to broil.

Line a baking sheet with parchment paper. Brush bread on both sides with oil. Place bread on the lined baking sheet and broil until one side is toasted, about 5 minutes, then remove from the oven. In a medium bowl, mash together the avocado, vinegar, and salt. Spread the avocado on the toasted side of the bread slices. Garnish with onion, sesame seeds, chives, and chili flakes. Optionally, you can also squeeze a lemon wedge over the toast. If using, add edible flowers before serving. Serve warm or at room temperature.

TIP The optional edible flowers can be found at farmers' markets, grocery stores, and online, or you can grow your own.

MAKES 4 SERVINGS

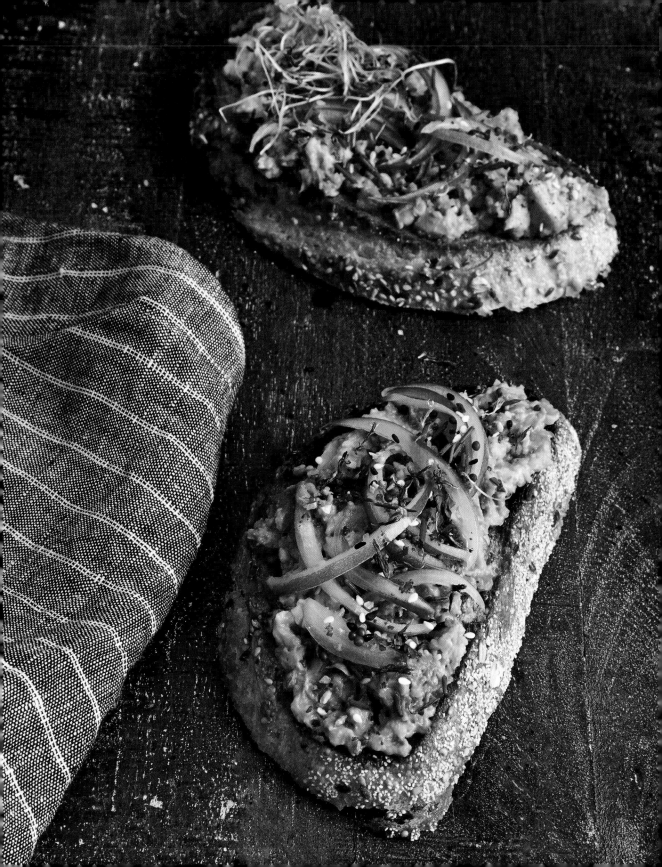

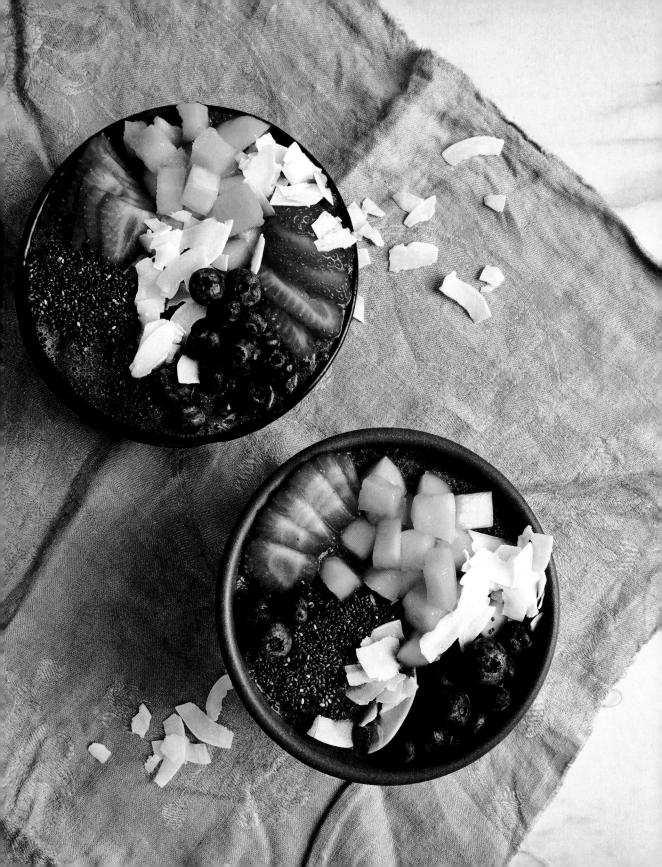

SUNRISE SMOOTHIE BOWL

Back in my early vegan days, before smoothie bowls were a thing, I used to make fruit soup. It was basically a very liquid smoothie that I used to pour in a bowl, top with things like granola, nuts, or fruit, and eat with a spoon. Twenty years later and smoothie bowls are everywhere. And although they're thicker than what I used to make, I still think my fruit soup is a contender. But whatever you call it, it makes for a delicious and ageless breakfast. The blueberries in this recipe help improve brain functioning and slow cognitive decline, and the chia seeds help make skin smoother and reduce wrinkling.

Place all filling ingredients in a blender with 3 cups water and blend until smooth and creamy. Spoon into serving bowls and add toppings in parallel rows. Serve immediately.

TIPS For a sweeter smoothie base, add 1 to 2 pitted Medjool dates.

You can also add Vanilla Cinnamon Granola with Almonds (page 94) as a topping for a great crunch.

MAKES 3-4 SERVINGS

FILLING
- 1 medium apple, cored and cut into chunks
- 1 ripe frozen banana, or 1 avocado, pitted
- 1 cup blueberries, fresh or frozen
- 1 tablespoon almond or cashew butter

TOPPINGS
- 1 mango, peeled and cubed
- 8 strawberries, thinly sliced
- 2 tablespoons unsweetened coconut flakes
- 1 teaspoon chia seeds

Chia Berry Breakfast Pudding

This is a tasty and nutritious breakfast that you can prep in individual jars a few days in advance to grab and go on busy mornings. The chia seeds provide protein and essential fiber, in addition to promoting smoother skin. And the three types of colorful berries provide ageless antioxidants that help promote brain functioning and slow cognitive decline.

½ cup chia seeds

1¾ cups unsweetened almond milk

1 tablespoon maple syrup or more to taste

¼ teaspoon vanilla extract (or the contents of 1 vanilla bean—see Tip)

Pinch sea salt

½ cup blackberries

¾ cup blueberries

¾ cup raspberries

2 tablespoons raw almonds, chopped

In a bowl, combine chia seeds, milk, maple syrup, vanilla, and salt. Cover, place in the refrigerator, and let sit for at least 2 hours or overnight. Serve topped with berries and almonds.

TIP To scrape the inside of a vanilla bean, use a paring knife to cut it lengthwise down the middle. Then use the dull side of the paring knife to gently scrape the insides of each half of the vanilla bean from tip to end.

MAKES 4 SERVINGS

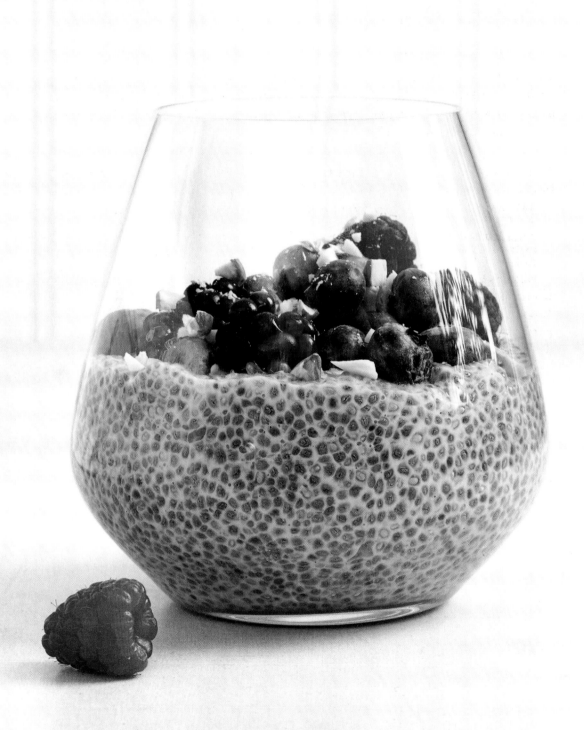

OVERNIGHT OATS
with PEAR AND PISTACHIOS

A delicious alternative to ordinary oatmeal, these fiber-rich and heart-healthy overnight oats offer an unexpected and delicious range of flavors. They also make mornings a whole lot easier. Just grab them from the fridge, add chopped pear and pistachios and a sprinkle of coconut flakes, and you have a nutritious breakfast in less than 5 minutes.

OATS

- 2 cups rolled oats
- 1 (13.5-ounce) can coconut milk (light)
- ½ cup unsweetened applesauce
- 1 tablespoon maple syrup
- ¼ teaspoon ground cardamom
- ⅛ teaspoon sea salt

TOPPINGS

- 1 pear, thinly sliced into strips
- 2 tablespoons unsweetened coconut flakes
- 2 tablespoons finely chopped pistachios

In a large bowl, combine the oats, milk, applesauce, maple syrup, cardamom, and salt. Cover and place in the refrigerator for 4 hours or overnight. To serve, place into individual serving bowls or cups and add the toppings.

MAKES 4 SERVINGS

AGELESS ANTIOXIDANTS   BRAIN BOOSTER   HEALTH IS IN THE HUE   LONGEVITY LOVER
PROTEIN DREAM   SMOOTH SKIN   STRONG BONES   SUPER GREENS   VISION MISSION

BANANA WALNUT MUFFINS

There's nothing better than the smell of banana muffins or bread baking in the oven. These muffins are super moist, with just the right amount of sweetness. I like to bake a dozen on the weekend so I can grab them for breakfast or a snack throughout the week. The walnuts add protein and essential omega oils and help make skin smoother.

Preheat oven to 350°F.

Line a muffin tin with paper cups or oil a muffin tin and set aside. In a large bowl, add flour, baking powder, baking soda, and salt and whisk until thoroughly combined. Stir in oat bran until combined. In a separate bowl, mash the bananas and add in oil, maple syrup, vanilla, and milk. Combine the banana mixture with the flour mixture and mix until just combined. Be sure not to over mix because that will lead to dry muffins. A few lumps here and there are fine. Fold in the ½ cup walnuts. Spoon batter into muffin cups or tin. Sprinkle remaining walnuts on top. Bake for 20 to 25 minutes, or until a toothpick inserted in the center comes out clean. Cool for at least 10 minutes or serve at room temperature. The muffins can be stored in an airtight container for about a week in the fridge and in a heavy-duty freezer bag in the freezer for 2 to 3 months.

MAKES 6 SERVINGS

1⅓ cups oat flour, sifted
1 teaspoon baking powder
1 teaspoon baking soda
½ teaspoon salt
½ cup oat bran
4 very ripe bananas
¼ cup extra-virgin coconut oil
¼ cup maple syrup
1 teaspoon vanilla extract
⅔ cup unsweetened almond milk
½ cup plus 2 tablespoons chopped walnuts

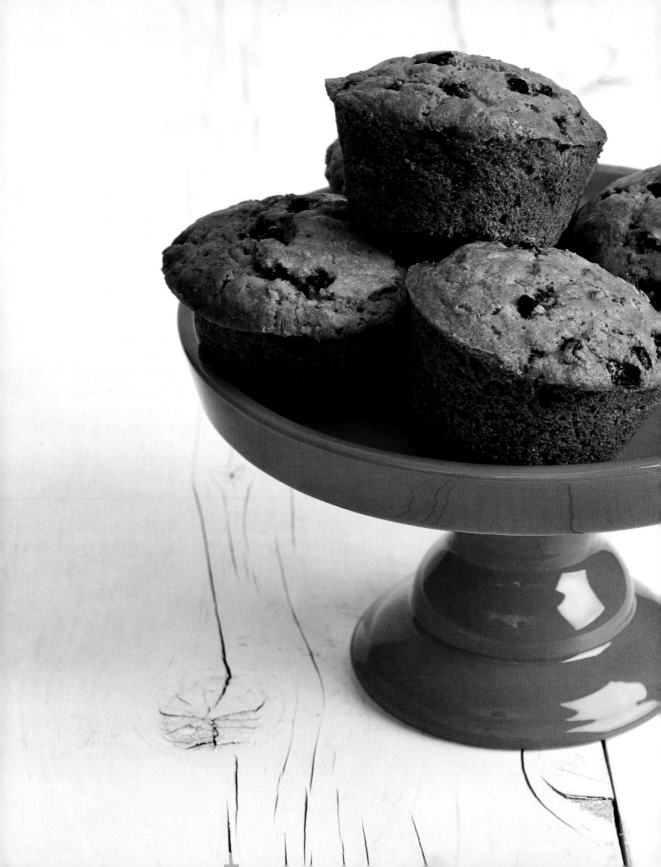

BLUEBERRY MUFFINS

Rich in heart-protecting, brain-boosting, and cancer-fighting antioxidants, berries are the healthiest fruits you can eat. So that's reason enough to double this recipe and have muffins on hand for breakfast or whenever you like. Blueberries are also naturally low in sugar, but you can decrease the amount of added maple syrup in this recipe to make these muffins even healthier.

Preheat oven to 350°F.

Line a muffin tin with paper cups or oil a muffin tin and set aside.

In a large bowl, add flour, baking soda, flaxseed meal, and salt and whisk until thoroughly combined. In a separate bowl, whisk together the milk, vinegar, syrup, oil, and vanilla. Combine the dry mixture with the wet mixture until just combined. Be sure not to over mix because that will lead to dry muffins. A few lumps here and there are fine. Fold in blueberries. Spoon batter into muffin cups or tin. Bake for 20 to 25 minutes, or until a toothpick inserted in the center comes out clean. Cool for at least 10 minutes or serve at room temperature. The muffins can be stored in an airtight container for about a week in the fridge and in a heavy-duty freezer bag in the freezer for 2 to 3 months.

MAKES 6 SERVINGS

1¾ cups whole wheat pastry flour, sifted

1½ teaspoons baking soda

¼ cup ground flaxseed meal

¼ teaspoon sea salt

1 cup unsweetened almond milk

1 tablespoon apple cider vinegar

½ cup maple syrup

¼ cup extra-virgin coconut oil

1 teaspoon vanilla extract

1 cup fresh blueberries

VANILLA CINNAMON GRANOLA
with ALMONDS

My mom loves making granola and giving it to family and friends. Everyone seems to love her recipe. The hint of coconut and cinnamon gives it a unique flavor, and it's healthier than most store-bought varieties. Try it with Coconut Cashew Milk (page 81).

⅓ cup extra-virgin coconut oil

¼ cup maple syrup

1 teaspoon vanilla extract

4 cups rolled oats

¼ cup oat bran (optional)

1 cup sunflower seeds

1 cup raw almonds

½ cup cashews

1 teaspoon cinnamon

Preheat oven to 275°F.

In a large bowl, combine oil, maple syrup, vanilla, and ⅛ cup water. In a separate bowl, combine the remaining ingredients. Add dry ingredients to liquid ingredients and use a spoon to mix well. Spread evenly onto two cookie sheets. Bake for 20 minutes and, using a spatula, turn over granola and bake for another 20 minutes. Serve warm or room temperature. Granola can be stored in an airtight container for 2 to 3 weeks in the fridge and up to 3 months in the freezer.

TIP Homemade granola is great to include in your essential stash of vegan snacks (which I talk about on page 43).

MAKES 6-8 SERVINGS

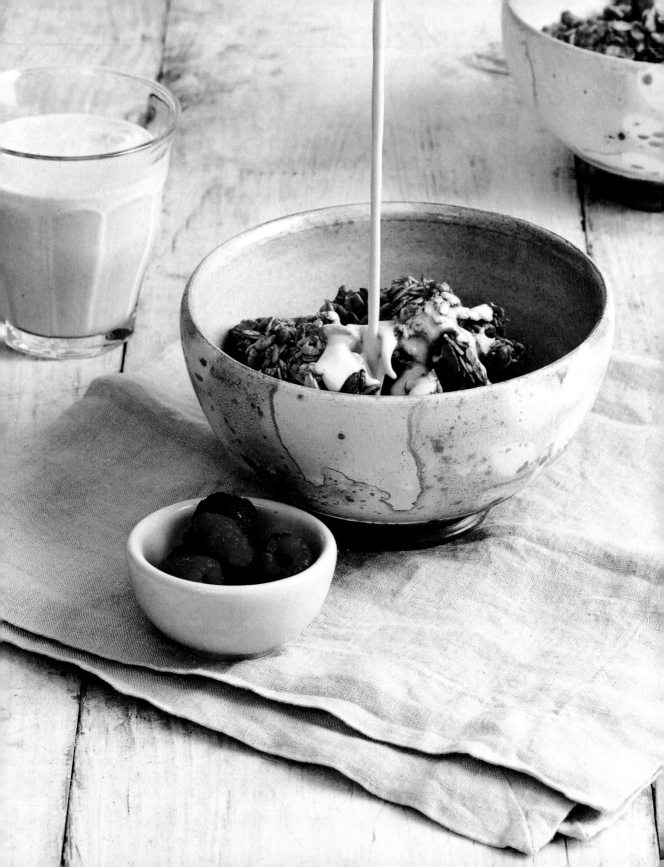

APPLE RAISIN GRANOLA
with PUMPKIN SEEDS

This apple variation of my mother's celebrated Vanilla Cinnamon Granola with Almonds also includes raisins, pumpkin seeds, cinnamon, and nutmeg. When eaten warm from the oven with Coconut Cashew Milk (page 81), it's reminiscent of an apple tart with ice cream—but for breakfast.

⅓ cup extra-virgin coconut oil

¼ cup maple syrup

1 teaspoon vanilla extract

4 cups rolled oats

1 large, firm apple, cored and diced

¼ cup oat bran (optional)

1 cup raw almonds

1 cup pumpkin seeds

½ cup cashews

½ cup raisins

½ cup unsweetened coconut flakes

1 teaspoon cinnamon

⅛ teaspoon nutmeg

Preheat oven to 275°F.

In a large bowl, combine oil, maple syrup, vanilla, and ⅛ cup water. In a separate bowl, combine the remaining ingredients. Add dry ingredients to liquid ingredients and use a spoon to mix well. Spread evenly onto two cookie sheets. Bake for 20 minutes and, using a spatula, turn over granola and bake for another 20 minutes. Serve warm or room temperature. Granola can be stored in an airtight container for 2 to 3 weeks in the fridge and up to 3 months in the freezer.

TIP Homemade granola is great to include in your essential stash of vegan snacks (which I talk about on page 43).

MAKES 6-8 SERVINGS

HOME FRIES

The magic ingredient in this recipe is thyme. This flavorful, aromatic herb elevates these home fries to something memorable. They're a must-have addition to your brunch menu.

In a large pot, bring 1½ cups water to a boil. Place a steamer insert in the pot, and steam potato slices for 10 to 15 minutes or until just tender, but not cooked completely. (Otherwise, they will fall apart when sautéing.) Set steamed potato slices aside.

In a large skillet, heat 1 tablespoon oil over medium heat. Add onions and sauté for 3 minutes or until translucent, stirring several times. Add the garlic and sauté for 1 to 2 more minutes, stirring constantly. Remove the onions and garlic from the pan and set aside. In the same skillet, heat the remaining oil over medium heat. Add the potato slices, onions, and garlic and sauté for 15 minutes or until golden brown. Stir in the thyme, salt, black pepper, and cayenne pepper (if using). Sauté for 1 to 2 more minutes. Serve hot.

MAKES 4 SERVINGS

- 4 medium red potatoes, peeled and thinly sliced (about ¼ inch thick)
- 3 tablespoons extra-virgin coconut oil
- 1 medium yellow onion, chopped
- 3 garlic cloves, finely chopped
- 2 teaspoons dried thyme
- ¼ teaspoon sea salt
- ⅛ teaspoon black pepper
- ⅛ teaspoon cayenne pepper (optional)

AGELESS ANTIOXIDANTS   BRAIN BOOSTER   HEALTH IS IN THE HUE   LONGEVITY LOVER
PROTEIN DREAM   SMOOTH SKIN   STRONG BONES   SUPER GREENS   VISION MISSION

97

MAPLE FRENCH TOAST
with STRAWBERRIES

This twist on French toast uses almond milk and bananas as the batter. I also like to use thick slices of fresh-baked or day-old whole-grain bread. It makes French toast that's golden brown with crispy edges on the outside and soft and moist on the inside. Topped with maple syrup, fresh fruit, and chopped nuts, it makes a wonderful centerpiece for Sunday brunch.

2 ripe bananas
⅔ cup unsweetened almond milk
1 teaspoon maple syrup
¼ teaspoon cinnamon
¼ teaspoon vanilla extract
2–3 tablespoons extra-virgin coconut oil
6 (½ to 1-inch-thick) slices whole-grain bread
Maple syrup, to taste
½ cup pecans, roughly chopped
2 cups strawberries, sliced

In a blender, add bananas, milk, maple syrup, cinnamon, and vanilla. Blend until thoroughly combined and smooth. Pour the batter into a large shallow bowl. Heat a large skillet with the 2 teaspoons of the oil over medium heat. Dip the bread into the batter and let it sit on each side for 15 to 20 seconds each to absorb some of the liquid. Let the excess liquid drip from the bread, then place the bread in the pan and cook on one side until golden brown, 2 to 3 minutes. Check and adjust the heat while the bread is cooking to make sure it doesn't burn. Gently flip the bread and cook the other side until golden brown, about 2 more minutes. Wipe out the pan, add about 2 teaspoons more oil, and repeat for the remaining slices of bread. Serve topped with maple syrup, pecans, and strawberries.

TIP You can place the cooked slices on a parchment paper–lined baking sheet in the oven at 200°F to keep them warm while you cook the rest.

MAKES 3-4 SERVINGS

AGELESS ANTIOXIDANTS BRAIN BOOSTER HEALTH IS IN THE HUE LONGEVITY LOVER
PROTEIN DREAM SMOOTH SKIN STRONG BONES SUPER GREENS VISION MISSION

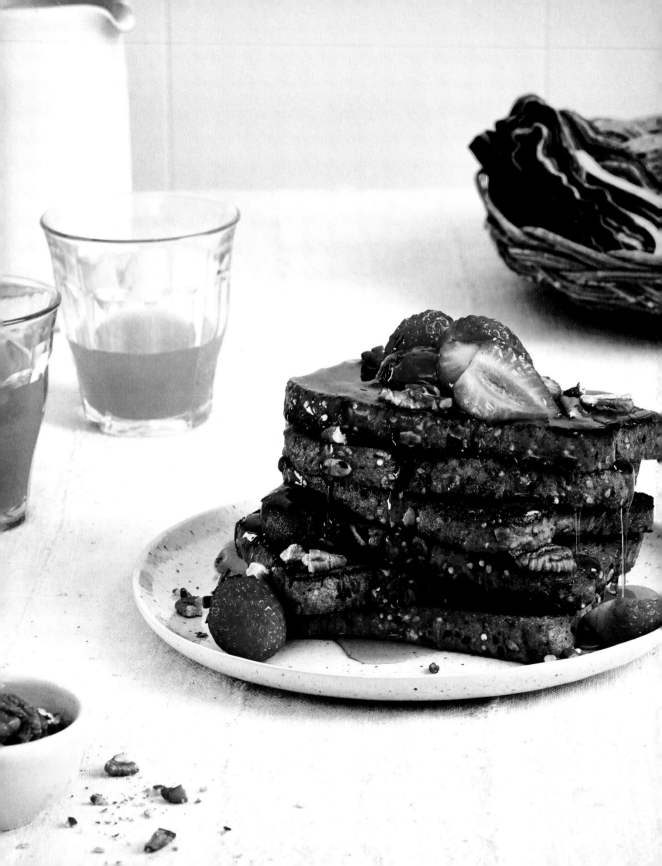

HOME-STYLE GRITS

Growing up, grits were always a part of our Sunday morning breakfasts. And because they're already vegan, they've kept their place on the table at our family's vegan brunches throughout the last thirty years. Simple, wholesome, and delicious, they taste great alongside Curried Tofu Scramble with Shiitake Mushrooms (page 101).

¼ teaspoon sea salt

¼ teaspoon extra-virgin coconut oil (optional)

½ cup yellow corn grits

Black pepper, to taste

1–2 teaspoons nutritional yeast (optional)

In a medium pot, bring 2 cups water, salt, and oil (if using) to a boil. Slowly add in grits while stirring. Reduce heat and simmer, stirring occasionally, until the water is absorbed and the grits are thick, about 10 minutes. Serve hot with black pepper and sprinkle with the nutritional yeast if you'd like a cheesy taste.

MAKES 3-4 SERVINGS

AGELESS ANTIOXIDANTS   BRAIN BOOSTER   HEALTH IS IN THE HUE   LONGEVITY LOVER
PROTEIN DREAM   SMOOTH SKIN   STRONG BONES   SUPER GREENS   VISION MISSION

CURRIED TOFU SCRAMBLE
with SHIITAKE MUSHROOMS

My mom's Tofu Scramble will make you forget about eggs! This protein-rich dish combines antioxidant-rich turmeric and cumin for a spicy curry flavor and a golden hue. She adds shiitake mushrooms for extra savory flavor and added nutrition. They help prevent inflammation and boost the immune system as we get older.

In a large skillet, heat the oil over medium heat. Stir in the onions and garlic and sauté until the onions are translucent, 3 to 5 minutes. Stir in the mushrooms and sauté until they are soft, about another 5 minutes. In a separate bowl, crumble tofu well with a fork. Add tofu to pan and stir. Then add remaining ingredients and sauté until water from tofu is cooked out, about 5 minutes, stirring constantly. Serve hot.

MAKES 3-4 SERVINGS

- 2 tablespoons extra-virgin olive oil
- 1 medium yellow onion, chopped
- 2 cloves fresh garlic, finely chopped
- 1 cup chopped shiitake (or Portobello) mushrooms
- 1 pound firm tofu
- ½ teaspoon basil
- 1 small hot red pepper, chopped
- 2 tablespoons nutritional yeast
- ½ teaspoon turmeric
- ⅛ teaspoon cumin
- 1 tablespoon low-sodium tamari
- 1 teaspoon dried parsley flakes

AVOCADO QUESADILLAS
with SALSA AND CASHEW SOUR CREAM

Quesadillas are among my favorite foods, and this recipe is no exception. Instead of cheese, they're filled with mushrooms, bell peppers, avocado, and salsa, and served with a dollop of homemade cashew sour cream. They make a wonderfully savory breakfast on their own or a hearty addition to Sunday brunch.

CASHEW SOUR CREAM

- 1 cup raw cashews
- 1 tablespoon freshly squeezed lemon juice (about ½ lemon)
- 1 teaspoon apple cider vinegar
- 1 garlic clove, peeled
- ⅛ teaspoon sea salt

QUESADILLA

- 1 tablespoon extra-virgin olive oil
- 1 small white onion, diced
- 2 garlic cloves, diced
- 1 large red bell pepper, seeds removed, thinly sliced
- 1 large orange bell pepper, seeds removed, thinly sliced
- 10 cremini mushrooms, thinly sliced
- ½ teaspoon sea salt
  - Black pepper, to taste
- 6 small or medium corn tortillas
- 2 large ripe avocados, pitted, and thinly sliced
  - Lime wedges, garnish (optional)

SALSA

- 6 tomatillos, sliced in half
- 2–3 serrano peppers (depending on how hot you like it)
- 1 small white onion, cut in quarters
- 3 garlic cloves, peeled
- 2 tablespoons fresh cilantro leaves, stems removed
  - Sea salt, to taste

CASHEW SOUR CREAM Place the cashews in a small bowl and cover by about ½ inch with boiling water for 30 minutes. Drain and rinse. Place the cashews in a high-speed blender with the lemon juice, vinegar, garlic, salt, and ¼ cup water. Blend on high until smooth, adding more water one tablespoon at a time, as needed to help blend. If desired, place sour cream in an airtight container and chill in the refrigerator for 30 minutes or more to thicken.

QUESADILLA Heat the oil in a large skillet over medium heat. Add the onion and garlic and sauté 2 minutes, until the onion is just slightly translucent. Add the bell peppers and sauté another 3 minutes. Add the mushrooms, salt, and pepper and sauté another 3 minutes. Remove the pan from the heat.

Heat a dry skillet on high to very hot. Add one tortilla and turn heat to medium. Heat the tortilla for about 30 seconds on each side and remove it from the pan. It should still be soft enough to fold in half without breaking.

SALSA Place all the ingredients and 1 tablespoon of water in blender and blend until smooth. Pour the salsa into a small bowl with a lid and keep it covered until serving to preserve its bright green color.

ASSEMBLE Divide the vegetable filling among the tortillas, placing the filling on one half of each tortilla. Top the filling with sliced avocados and salsa. Fold the tortillas in half and serve with cashew sour cream on the side. Garnish with lime wedges, if desired.

MAKES 6 SERVINGS

6

Snacks & Bites

One of the things we love most about these healthy snacks and bites, besides how good they taste, is how versatile they are. They're great as stand-alone foods to munch on between meals, and they also make great appetizers for casual get-togethers, especially Stuffed Mushrooms, Summer Rolls, and Artichoke Dip with Pita Chips. And for more options, Crunchy Roasted Chickpeas, Sweet and Spicy Oven-Toasted Almonds, and Crispy Tofu Bites can be tossed into everything from salads to soups to stir-fries.

Crunchy Roasted Chickpeas

Sweet and Spicy Oven-Toasted Almonds

Tahini Oat Banana Bites

Crispy Tofu Bites

Artichoke Dip with Pita Chips

Sweet Pea Hummus

Summer Rolls

Stuffed Mushrooms

CRUNCHY
ROASTED CHICKPEAS

Craving something savory and spicy? Don't reach for the chips, reach for this super tasty and protein-packed snack. You can eat these chickpeas on their own or add them as a topping on salads and soups, instead of croutons. Simple to make and so satisfying to eat, you'll definitely want to roast a double or triple batch.

1 tablespoon extra-virgin olive oil

1 teaspoon all-purpose dried herbs and vegetables seasoning blend

½ teaspoon turmeric

¼ teaspoon cayenne pepper

⅛ teaspoon sea salt, or to taste

1 (15-ounce) can chickpeas, drained, rinsed, and thoroughly patted dry

Preheat oven to 400ºF.

Line a baking sheet with parchment paper and set aside. In a medium bowl, combine the oil, seasoning blend, turmeric, cayenne pepper, and salt. Add the chickpeas and mix well, until all the chickpeas are coated. Place the chickpeas on the lined baking sheet. Bake until the outside is crispy, 30 to 40 minutes, shaking the tray to toss the chickpeas about halfway through. Then turn off the oven and leave the chickpeas inside until the oven cools. This will dehydrate the chickpeas and make them crunchy. You can also leave the chickpeas in the oven overnight. If you don't want the chickpeas to be that crunchy, you can take them out of the oven immediately after baking and serve them warm or let them cool. They'll be crispy and chewy, rather than crunchy. Either way, serve the chickpeas at room temperature. Store them in an airtight container outside of the fridge for up to 2 weeks, if they last that long!

MAKES 4 SERVINGS

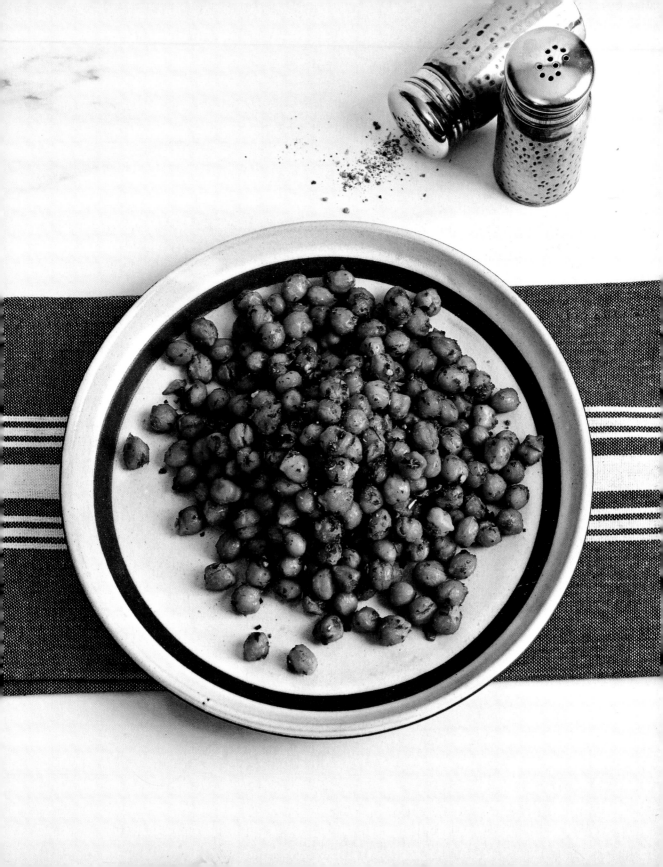

Oven-Toasted Almonds

If you like a little sweetness with your spice and crunch, these almonds will do the trick. Versatile and delicious, they can be eaten alone as a snack or tossed in just about anything, from salads to stir-fries. Almonds are high in calcium, which helps strengthen bones, and rich in vitamin E, which protects the body from free-radical damage that can result in premature aging.

1 cup raw almonds
2 teaspoons maple syrup
  Cayenne pepper, to taste
¼ teaspoon sea salt (or more, to taste)

Preheat oven to 200°F.

In a large bowl, combine all the ingredients with ¼ teaspoon water. Line a baking sheet with parchment paper and place nuts on the baking sheet. Bake until the nuts are toasted and the liquid is absorbed, about 4 hours, or nuts can be left in the oven overnight at 200°F, about 8 hours. Serve immediately or store in an airtight container outside of the fridge for up to 1 week.

MAKES 4 SERVINGS

TAHINI OAT BANANA BITES

These bites are great to have on hand when you want something quick, light, and nutritious to fuel your morning workout. I like to grab a couple to energize my early morning walks. They're also ideal when you want a bite of something sweet and nutritious after dinner during the week. Tahini is a rich source of calcium and phosphorous, which help strengthen bones and teeth.

Preheat oven to 350°F.

Line a baking sheet with parchment paper and set aside. In a medium bowl, combine oats and banana until a sticky mixture is formed. Add remaining ingredients and combine. Pack mixture into a tablespoon measure and drop onto the lined baking sheet. You may need to use a knife to help scoop out the mixture. Bake for 10 to 12 minutes, or until oats turn golden brown. Serve warm or at room temperature. Store in an airtight container inside or outside of the fridge for up to 1 week.

TIPS These bites are not intended to be very sweet, but you can add ½ teaspoon of maple syrup, if desired.

1 tablespoon of almond, cashew, or other nut butter can be substituted for the tahini.

MAKES ABOUT 15-20 BITES

1 cup rolled oats

1 ripe large banana, or 1½ medium bananas, mashed

½ cup unsweetened shredded coconut

¼ cup raisins (optional)

1 tablespoon tahini

½ teaspoon vanilla extract

¼ teaspoon cinnamon

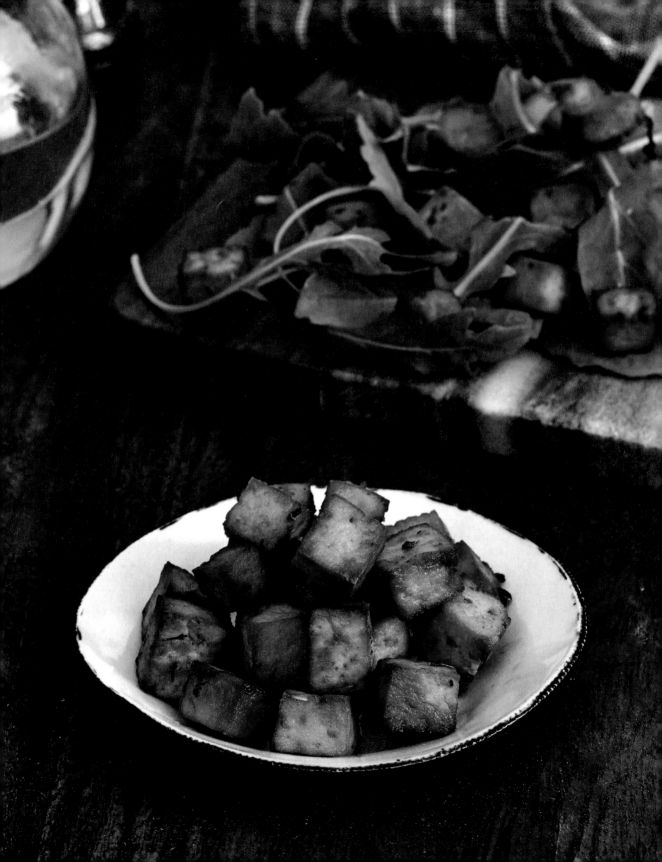

CRISPY TOFU BITES

The beauty of these protein-hearty bites is that they're oven-baked, so they give you crispy tofu without frying. The marinade makes them spicy, and they bake up deliciously firm and chewy. They can be eaten as they are, as a hot or cold snack, or added to salads, stir-fries, pastas, wraps ... you name it!

Preheat oven to 400°F.

In a large bowl, whisk together oil and coconut aminos with 2 tablespoons water. Whisk in remaining seasonings. Place tofu cubes in the bowl and gently fold, making sure all the cubes are coated. Sprinkle on nutritional yeast and gently fold, making sure all the cubes are coated. Spread the cubes onto the baking sheet. Bake for 15 minutes and then flip cubes. I use steel tongs or a fork to turn over each cube. Bake for 10 more minutes. Taste and adjust seasonings, as needed. Serve hot or at room temperature.

TIP Tempeh chopped in cubes can be used instead of tofu.

MAKES 4 SERVINGS

1 tablespoon extra-virgin olive or sesame oil

1 tablespoon coconut aminos or low-sodium tamari

¼ teaspoon turmeric

¼ teaspoon cayenne pepper

½ teaspoon all-purpose dried herbs and vegetables seasoning blend

Dash hot sauce, to taste

1 block extra-firm tofu, cut into ½-inch cubes

2 tablespoons nutritional yeast

ARTICHOKE DIP
with PITA CHIPS

The traditional version of this dish is very heavy with dairy cheese and mayo. This vegan version eliminates the cholesterol, cuts down on the fat, keeps all the flavor, and adds an ageless antioxidant boost with the inclusion of vision-protecting spinach. I like this dip warm right from the oven. The toasted pita chips, with just a touch of salt and olive oil, are the perfect spoons.

DIP

- ¾ cup raw cashews
- ¾ cup unsweetened almond milk
- 3 tablespoons freshly squeezed lemon juice (about 1½ lemons)
- 2 cloves raw or roasted garlic, roughly chopped
- 1 tablespoon nutritional yeast
- 1 teaspoon whole-grain mustard
- 2 (9-ounce) jars of artichoke hearts (from jars packed with water, thoroughly drained)
- 2 cups fresh spinach
- ¼ teaspoon sea salt
   Freshly ground black pepper, to taste

PITA CHIPS

- 2 (6-inch) whole-grain pita breads, cut into 12 smaller pieces (24 pieces total)
- 1 tablespoon extra-virgin olive oil
- ¼ teaspoon sea salt

DIP Preheat oven to 425°F.

Place cashews, milk, lemon juice, garlic, nutritional yeast, and mustard in a food processor and process until very smooth. Add artichoke hearts, spinach, salt, and pepper and pulse the food processor on and off until the mixture is combined but some chunks of artichoke and spinach remain. Place in a large baking dish, and bake for 20 minutes. Serve immediately with pita chips.

CHIPS Preheat oven to 350°F.

Place the pita pieces in a single layer on a baking sheet. Brush one side of the pita pieces with oil. Sprinkle with sea salt. Bake until crispy, about 15 minutes. Chips and dip can be served warm or at room temperature.

MAKES 4-6 SERVINGS

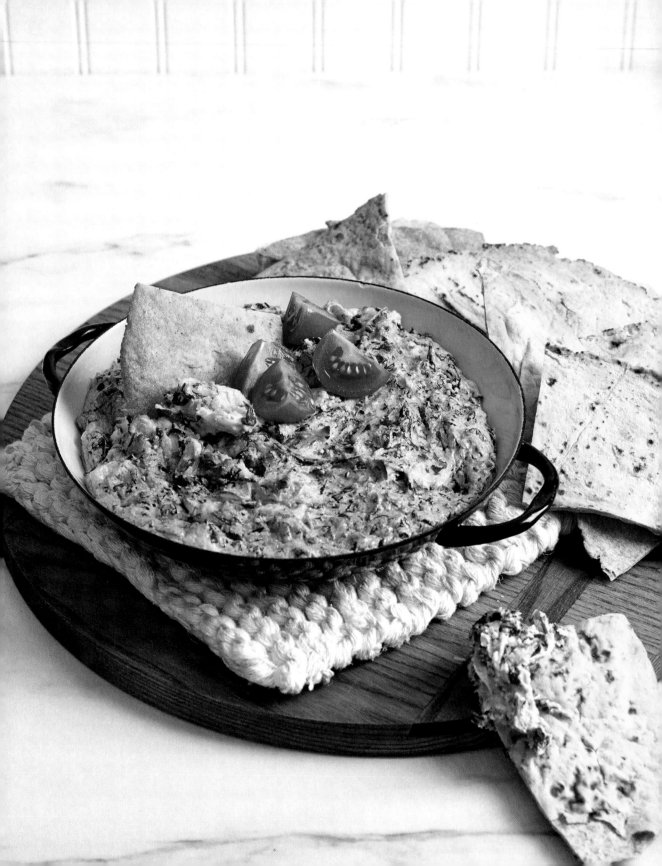

Sweet Pea Hummus

This hummus is made from sweet green peas instead of chickpeas. It's a light, vibrant change of pace but with all the flavor and creaminess of traditional hummus. And the ageless antioxidants in peas help reduce premature wrinkling of the skin, especially around the eyes.

1 cup cooked peas (if fresh, cook in boiling water for 2 minutes; if frozen, cook according to package instructions; take care not to overcook)

¼ cup cilantro leaves

1½ tablespoons tahini

2 tablespoons freshly squeezed lemon juice (about 1 lemon)

1 garlic clove, fresh or roasted, finely chopped

¼ teaspoon sea salt

Combine all the ingredients in a food processor and process for 30 to 40 seconds. Serve with fresh-cut veggies or toasted pita chips (see recipe on page 112).

MAKES 4 SERVINGS

Summer Rolls

These colorful, heart-healthy, mostly raw versions of deep-fried spring rolls are perfect for a light lunch during hot summer months.

BLACK RICE In a large pot, bring black rice and ¾ cup plus 2 tablespoons water to a boil. Reduce the heat, cover, and simmer for 45 minutes. Remove from the heat and let sit for 10 minutes, covered, to finish cooking. In a medium bowl, combine the black rice, sesame oil, and salt.

SAUCE In a blender, combine the sauce ingredients and ¼ cup water.

ASSEMBLE Fill a pie dish with water. Take a single sheet of rice paper and soak in water for 20 seconds, remove from water, pat dry to remove excess water, and lay on a clean, dry cutting board. Place one-quarter of the black rice, bell pepper, cucumbers, avocado, carrot, and micro greens in rows on the third of the wrapper closest to you. Leave a half inch on each end empty. Tightly roll up the wrapper, tucking the ends in. Serve whole or sliced in half with sauce.

TIP Brown rice spring roll wrappers are available in some national grocery store chains and can be ordered online.

MAKES 6-8 SERVINGS

BLACK RICE
- ½ cup black rice
- 1 tablespoon sesame oil
- ¼ teaspoon sea salt

SAUCE
- ⅓ cup peanut butter
- 2 tablespoons rice vinegar
- 1 tablespoon coconut aminos or low-sodium tamari
- 1 teaspoon peeled and grated ginger

ROLLS
- 6–8 brown rice spring roll wrappers
- 1 red bell pepper, seeds removed, thinly sliced
- 1 cup very thinly sliced cucumbers (about 1 medium cucumber)
- 1 avocado, pitted and sliced into eight pieces
- ½ cup grated carrot (about 1 medium carrot)
- 1 cup micro greens

STUFFED MUSHROOMS

These stuffed mushrooms are piled high with nutritious black rice and topped with a cheesy crumble made from nutritional yeast and cashews. Black rice is high in anthocyanidins, the plant pigment that gives these foods their rich color and powerful anti-aging properties, which include improving brain functioning and slowing cognitive decline.

MUSHROOMS

- 10 large white or cremini mushrooms, stems removed
- 1½ tablespoons extra-virgin olive oil
- ¼ teaspoon sea salt

SEASONING

- 3 tablespoons nutritional yeast
- ½ cup cashew pieces
- ¼ teaspoon sea salt
  Cayenne pepper, to taste

FILLING

- ½ cup cooked black rice or other whole grain, such as bulgur or brown rice
- 1 garlic clove, finely chopped
- 1 tablespoon extra-virgin olive oil
- ½ teaspoon chopped fresh thyme leaves
- ¼ teaspoon sea salt
  Freshly ground black pepper, to taste
  Micro greens, garnish (optional)

MUSHROOMS Preheat oven to 375°F.

Line a baking sheet with parchment paper and set aside. In a large bowl, add mushrooms and coat the outside of the mushrooms with oil and salt. Place on the lined baking sheet with mushroom interiors facing up. Bake for 10 minutes.

SEASONING While mushrooms are cooking, put the seasoning ingredients in a food processor and pulse on and off about five times, until the cashews are processed to very small chunks.

FILLING In a bowl, combine half of the seasoning mixture, black rice, garlic, oil, thyme, salt, and pepper.

ASSEMBLE Remove the mushrooms from the oven. Add any water from the mushrooms to the rice mixture. Using your fingers, stuff the mushrooms high with the rice mixture, then top with the remaining seasoning mixture. Bake for 15 more minutes. Garnish with micro greens, if desired.

MAKES 2-4 SERVINGS

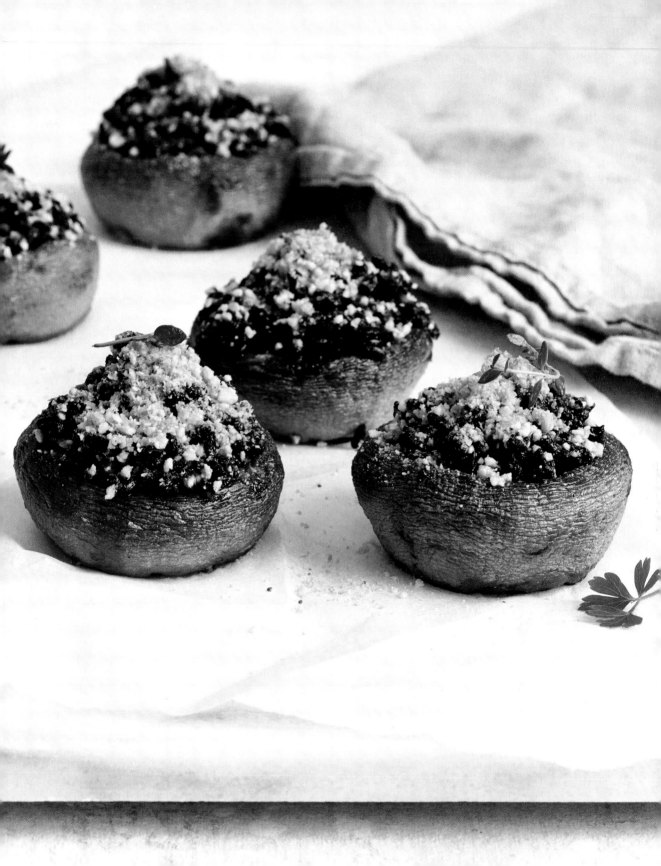

Soups & Sides

There's nothing quite like a bowl of hot soup and a slice of rustic bread on a cold winter's day. It makes life cozy. All of the soups in this chapter are heart-warming and delicious, like Thai Coconut Curry Soup, Navy Bean and Kale Soup, and Lemongrass Noodle Soup. And the side dishes are stars in their own right, including rich and creamy Mac and Cheese, spicy Cajun Quinoa with Okra and Tomato, and fragrant Chana Masala.

Thai Coconut Curry Soup

Yellow Split Pea Soup with Red Onion

Farro with Shiitake Mushrooms

Lemongrass Noodle Soup

Peanut Soup with Collards

Navy Bean and Kale Soup

Southern-Style Cornbread

Curried Lentil Soup with Carrots and Rosemary

Saffron Rice

Baked Sweet Potato Fries with Garlic and Truffle Oil

Herbed Potato Salad

Spiced and Sautéed Sweet Potatoes

Black-Eyed Peas Salad

Cajun Quinoa with Okra and Tomato

Chana Masala

Mac and Cheese

Black Bean Soup with Avocado and Cashew Sour Cream

THAI COCONUT CURRY SOUP

This is one of my favorite soups. The curry and coconut milk combination makes this dish spicy, creamy, and delicious. And the sauce is a great base for most any colorful vegetables, so you can easily tweak this recipe to include your own favorites. It's a great example of a nutritious Health Is in the Hue dish. It's also simple to prepare, which makes it perfect for weeknight dinners.

CURRY PASTE

- 2 garlic cloves
- 1 tablespoon peeled and grated ginger
- 2 tomatoes, diced
- 1 jalapeño, roughly chopped (see Tip)
- 1 tablespoon ground coriander
- 2 teaspoons ground cumin
- ½ teaspoon turmeric
- ¼ teaspoon black pepper

NOODLES

- 1 (8-ounce) package of thin brown rice Asian noodles, cooked according to package instructions
- 1 tablespoon extra-virgin coconut oil
- ½ teaspoon sea salt

SOUP

- 1 tablespoon extra-virgin coconut oil
- ½ medium yellow onion, thinly sliced
- 1 (13.5-ounce) can coconut milk (light or regular)
- 2 teaspoons sea salt
- 2 cups snow peas or sugar snap peas
- 2 cups thinly sliced carrots (cut into rounds)
- 2 cups broccoli florets

GARNISH

- 1 lime, sliced into 6 wedges
- 1 cup basil leaves, loosely packed
  Red pepper flakes, to taste

CURRY PASTE In a blender, combine the garlic, ginger, tomatoes, jalapeño, coriander, cumin, turmeric, and black pepper.

NOODLES In a medium bowl, combine the noodles with oil and salt.

SOUP In a large soup pot, heat the oil over medium heat. Stir in the onions, and sauté until the onions are translucent, 3 to 5 minutes. Add the coconut milk, 1 cup water, salt, and curry paste. Reduce the heat to low and simmer for 15 minutes. Add snow peas, carrots, and broccoli and simmer for 5 minutes. Turn off the heat and stir in the noodles. Top each serving with a fresh lime for squeezing, basil, and pepper flakes. This soup can be stored in the fridge up to 2 days in an airtight container.

TIP A fresh pepper's heat depends on the variety and the size. For very spicy dishes, use one habañero; for medium, use one to two jalapeños, and for mild, use one poblano or one Anaheim. Much of the heat is in the seeds, so clean those out well if you want to temper the heat a bit. Remember to wear gloves when seeding hot peppers.

MAKES 6 SERVINGS

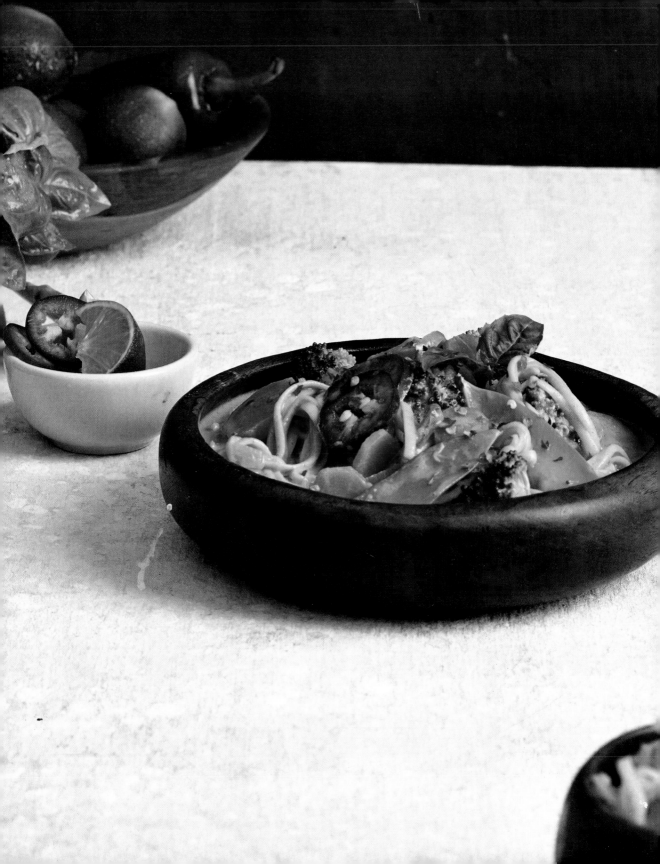

YELLOW SPLIT PEA SOUP
with RED ONION

Split peas are high in protein and fiber, they cook fast (no need for presoaking), and they're easily digested. The antioxidant-rich carrots, herbs, and spices dial up the flavor of this soup without being overpowering. Enjoy it with toasted rustic bread and a side salad, like Arugula Salad with Walnuts and Caesar Dressing (page 148).

SOUP

- 1 tablespoon extra-virgin olive oil
- ½ medium red onion, thinly sliced
- 2 garlic cloves, finely chopped
- 1½ cups dried yellow split peas, rinsed
- 1 cup chopped carrot (about 1 medium carrot)
- 1 tablespoon thyme
- 2¼ teaspoons sea salt, or more to taste
- Freshly ground black pepper, to taste

GARNISH

- ½ medium red onion, cut into ¼-inch thick rings
- 1 tablespoon extra-virgin olive oil
- ¼ teaspoon sea salt
- 2 tablespoons chopped dill

SOUP Preheat oven to broil.

In a large soup pot, heat the oil over medium heat. Stir in the onions and garlic and sauté until the onions are translucent, 3 to 5 minutes. Add 6 cups water, split peas, carrots, thyme, salt, and pepper and bring to a boil. Reduce the heat to low, cover, and simmer for 30 minutes. Put 2 cups of the soup in a blender and blend until smooth. Return the puréed soup to the chunky soup in the pot and combine.

GARNISH While the soup is cooking, place the onion rings in a medium bowl and coat with oil and salt. Place on a baking sheet lined with parchment paper and broil until onions turn brown, turn over with a spatula, and repeat on the other side, about 3 minutes on each side. Garnish soup with the onion rings and dill. This soup freezes well in airtight containers, so it's one that can be made in large batches and stored for lunch and dinner during the week.

MAKES 6 SERVINGS

FARRO
with SHIITAKE MUSHROOMS

Farro is a whole grain derived from wheat. If it's not a regular part of your whole grains repertoire, it should be. Farro has a firm chewiness similar to barley when cooked, which gives it a lovely texture and mouthfeel. This recipe pairs farro with shiitake mushrooms for a rich and earthy flavor and nutrition boost—shiitakes help strengthen the immune system and prevent inflammation. Celery is also a nutrition powerhouse in this dish—the anti-inflammatory compound luteolin in celery helps protect against brain inflammation that can lead to dementia.

Preheat oven to broil.

Place 5 cups water in a 3-quart pan and bring to a boil. Add the farro to the boiling water and bring to a boil again. Reduce the heat, cover, and simmer until tender, about 20 minutes. Taste the farro to test for tenderness. Remove the pot from the heat. Drain and rinse the farro and set aside.

Place the mushrooms in a bowl and coat with 1½ teaspoons of the oil and ¼ teaspoon of the salt. Place the mushrooms on a baking sheet lined with parchment paper and broil until the tips of the mushrooms turn brown, about 5 minutes. The exact timing will depend on the strength of your broiler and how close the baking sheet is to the heat source.

In a large bowl, combine the farro, mushrooms, celery, the remaining 1½ teaspoons oil, chives, the remaining ½ teaspoon of salt, and pepper. Taste and adjust the seasonings, as desired. Serve hot or at room temperature.

TIP Do not use instant or quick-cooking farro in this recipe, as it will not cook the same way as regular dry farro.

MAKES 4 SERVINGS

1½ cups dry farro, rinsed and drained

4 cups shiitake mushrooms, thinly sliced (about 16 medium mushrooms)

1 tablespoon extra-virgin olive oil

¾ teaspoon sea salt

3 stalks celery, thinly sliced

10 chives, cut into ½-inch pieces

Freshly ground black pepper, to taste

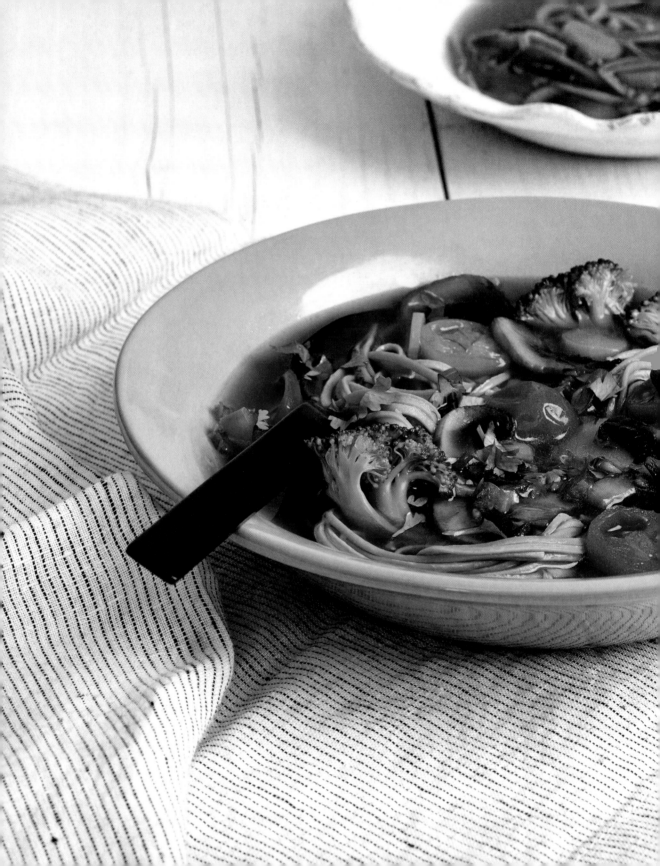

LEMONGRASS NOODLE SOUP

If lemongrass is new to you, it's an aromatic plant with stalks that smell like lemon and are used as flavoring. Lemongrass stalks are widely available in mass market grocery stores, health food stores, and specialty stores. Their antioxidant properties help prevent free-radical damage that can increase the risk for chronic diseases, such as heart disease and cancer. This soup is citrusy, sweet, tangy, and spicy, and the fettuccine is thick and chewy. It's chock-full of flavor and texture.

In a large soup pot, heat the oil over medium heat. Stir in the garlic and ginger and sauté until fragrant, about 1 minute. Add 4 cups water, lemongrass, mushrooms, tomatoes, celery, and chile and bring to a boil. Reduce the heat to low, cover, and simmer for 20 minutes. Add the carrot, broccoli, tamari, and salt and return to a boil. As soon as it boils, remove from heat. To serve, remove the pieces of lemongrass, stir in the fettuccine and lime juice, and garnish with cilantro.

TIP Explore brand makes the pasta called for in this recipe and it's available at healthier food stores and online. Other whole-grain noodles can be easily substituted, such as soba, angel hair, or spaghetti noodles.

MAKES 4 SERVINGS

1 tablespoon extra-virgin olive oil

2 garlic cloves, finely chopped

2 teaspoons peeled and finely chopped ginger

4 stalks lemongrass, cut in half lengthwise

12 mushrooms, sliced (about 2 cups)

10 cherry tomatoes, halved (about 1 cup)

1 stalk celery, cut into ⅛-inch slices

1 serrano chile, chopped

1 medium carrot, cut into ⅛-inch slices

2 cups broccoli florets

2 tablespoons low-sodium tamari

¾ teaspoon sea salt

1 (7-ounce) package edamame and mung bean fettuccine, cooked according to package instructions

1 tablespoon freshly squeezed lime juice (about ½ lime)

¼ cup chopped cilantro leaves, for garnish

PEANUT SOUP
with COLLARDS

This creamy, protein-rich soup is made with a simple medley of crunchy peanut butter, collard greens, and tomatoes. Hearty and healthy (but not heavy), this soup can be eaten on its own or combined with rice or quinoa for added texture and protein. As super-nutritious dark leafy greens, collards are high in vitamin A, which supports vision functioning, and vitamin K, which helps keep bones strong.

1 tablespoon extra-virgin coconut oil

1 medium yellow onion, sliced

2 tablespoons peeled and grated ginger

3 garlic cloves, finely chopped

1 cup crunchy, unsalted, dry-roasted peanut butter

½ bunch collard greens, ribs removed and leaves thinly sliced

2 medium tomatoes, chopped

1 tablespoon sea salt

Freshly ground black pepper, to taste

Red pepper flakes, to taste

In a large soup pot, heat the oil over medium heat. Stir in the onions, ginger, and garlic and sauté until the onions are translucent, 3 to 5 minutes. Add 3 cups water and the peanut butter and stir until thoroughly incorporated. Add the collard greens, tomatoes, salt, pepper, and pepper flakes. Reduce the heat to low, cover, and simmer until the collard greens are tender and the soup is thick, about 20 minutes. Taste and season again with salt, pepper, and red pepper, to taste. Serve hot. This soup can be stored in the fridge up to 2 days in an airtight container.

MAKES 4 SERVINGS

Navy Bean and Kale Soup

This soup is loaded with fiber, protein, vision-protecting lutein, and bone-strengthening calcium and vitamin K, among other nutrients. It's also light, simple, and flavorful, and is one of my favorite go-to recipes.

In a large soup pot, heat the oil over medium heat. Stir in the onions and garlic, and sauté until the onions are translucent, 3 to 5 minutes, stirring often. Add the tomatoes, 4 cups water, salt, and pepper. Reduce the heat to low, cover, and simmer for 10 minutes. Add the fennel, kale, and beans. Simmer until the kale is tender, about 15 minutes. Serve hot with a thick slice of crusty bread. This soup can be stored in the fridge up to 2 days in an airtight container.

MAKES 6 SERVINGS

1 tablespoon extra-virgin olive oil

1 medium yellow onion, thinly sliced

2 garlic cloves, finely chopped

4 medium tomatoes, diced

1½ teaspoons sea salt

Freshly ground pepper, to taste

2 cups thinly sliced fennel bulb, core removed (about 1 large bulb)

4 cups kale, stems removed and greens thinly sliced

2 cups precooked navy beans, or about 1½ (15-ounce) cans

SOUTHERN-STYLE CORNBREAD

This classic cornbread is light and mildly sweet, with a perfectly crumbly texture. It's so easy to make, you can whip it up quickly to eat with any of the delectable soups in this chapter. And you'll be getting the ageless antioxidant benefit of corn that helps reduce premature wrinkling of the skin.

¼ cup plus 1 tablespoon safflower oil, grapeseed oil, or other nonflavored oil

1½ cups yellow cornmeal

1¼ cups whole wheat pastry flour, sifted

2 teaspoons baking powder

½ teaspoon sea salt

1½ cups unsweetened soy milk or almond milk

1 tablespoon apple cider vinegar

⅓ cup maple syrup

Preheat oven to 350ºF.

Use 1 tablespoon of the oil to grease a 13 x 9-inch baking dish. In a medium bowl, combine cornmeal, flour, baking powder, and salt. In a separate bowl, combine milk, vinegar, maple syrup, and the remaining oil. Stir the wet mixture into the flour mixture. Pour batter into the baking dish and bake for 45 minutes or until a fork inserted in the center comes out clean. Serve warm or at room temperature. Cornbread can be frozen in a heavy-duty freezer bag for up to 3 months.

MAKES 8-10 SERVINGS

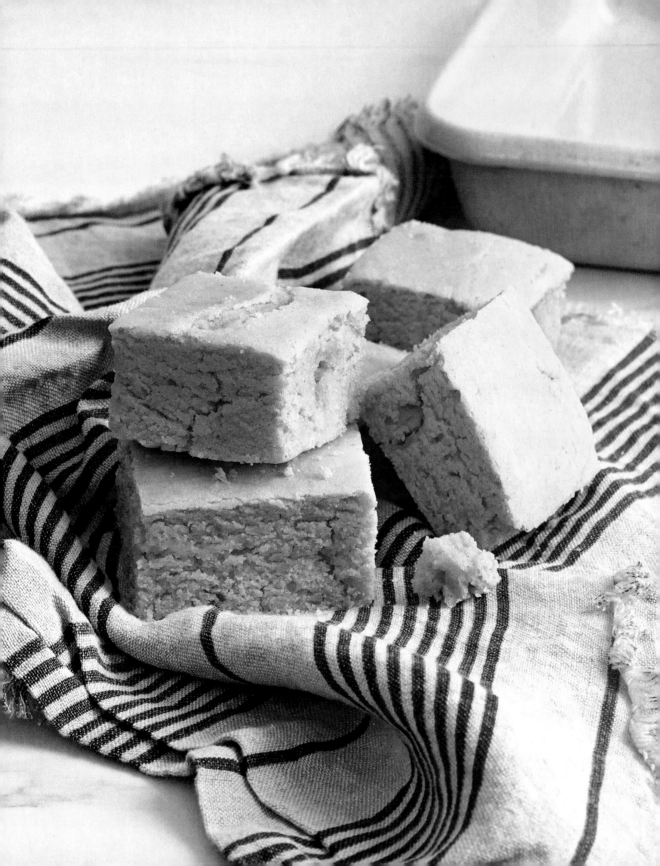

CURRIED LENTIL SOUP
with CARROTS AND ROSEMARY

My mom came up with this recipe because she wanted to create a lentil soup that was as good as the one at her favorite vegan restaurant. It's light, heart-healthy, and comforting. And the mix of seasonings and vegetables add richness and depth of flavor. The turmeric, rosemary, and celery also help improve cognitive functioning. And the lentils are among the most potent plant-based sources of cholesterol-lowering fiber as well as protein. It's the perfect soup to make in large batches over the weekend and eat for lunch and dinner throughout the week.

1½ cups dried green lentils, rinsed and drained

1 tablespoon extra-virgin olive oil

1 medium yellow onion, chopped

1 large carrot, chopped

1 stalk celery, chopped

2 garlic cloves, chopped

1 medium red or gold potato, chopped

1 teaspoon barley miso

1 teaspoon curry powder

½ teaspoon low-sodium tamari

½ teaspoon basil

½ teaspoon rosemary

⅛ teaspoon turmeric

⅛ teaspoon cayenne

⅛ teaspoon sea salt

Place the lentils and 4 cups water in a large pot and simmer until tender (about 1 hour). In a skillet, heat the oil and sauté the onions, carrots, celery, garlic, and potatoes. About 10 minutes before the lentils are done, add the sautéed vegetables and remaining ingredients to the lentils and continue cooking until lentils are tender. Serve hot. This soup freezes well for batch cooking.

MAKES 8 SERVINGS

AGELESS ANTIOXIDANTS   BRAIN BOOSTER   HEALTH IS IN THE HUE   LONGEVITY LOVER
PROTEIN DREAM   SMOOTH SKIN   STRONG BONES   SUPER GREENS   VISION MISSION

SAFFRON RICE

The beautiful burnt-orange color of saffron gives this rice a pretty and festive golden yellow hue when cooked. But even better, it gives the long-grain brown rice in this recipe a deliciously subtle floral flavor and aroma that's truly unique. This dish pairs well with Chana Masala (page 141), Colorful Kebab (page 179), and Three-Bean Chili (page 204).

In a medium saucepan with a tight-fitting lid, heat the oil over medium heat. Stir in the onions and garlic and sauté until the onions are translucent, 3 to 5 minutes. Add saffron and paprika and sauté for 30 seconds, and then add 2¼ cups water and salt. Bring to a boil and stir. Add the rice, reduce the heat to low, cover, and simmer for 40 minutes, or until the water is absorbed. Remove from the heat and let sit with the lid on for 10 minutes to finish cooking. To serve, fluff the rice with a fork and mix in the parsley.

TIP A quarter teaspoon of turmeric can be substituted for the saffron.

MAKES 4 SERVINGS

1 tablespoon extra-virgin olive oil

¼ onion, finely chopped

2 garlic cloves, finely chopped

1 teaspoon saffron or 4 pinches saffron threads

½ teaspoon smoked paprika

¾ teaspoon sea salt

1 cup long-grain brown rice

¼ cup chopped flat-leaf parsley

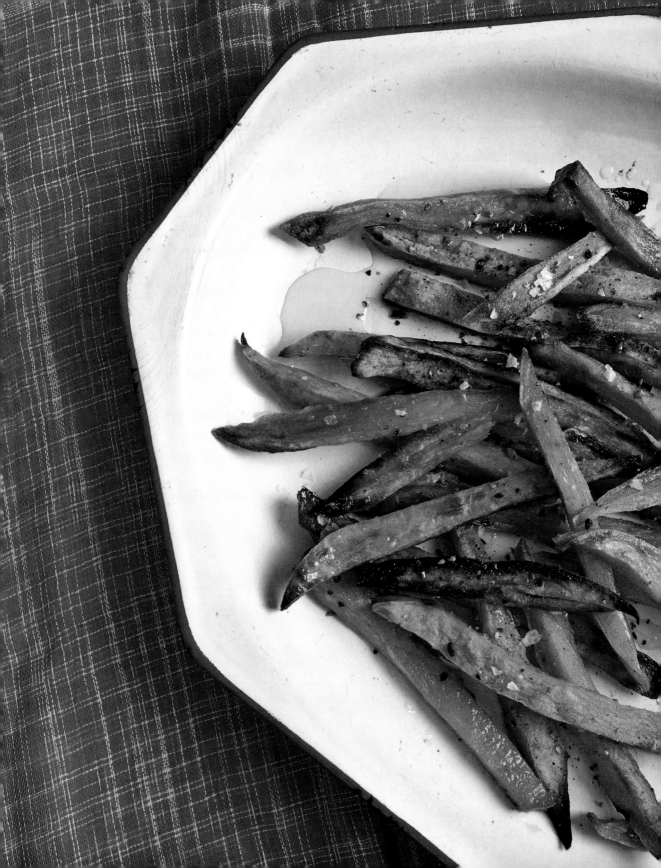

BAKED SWEET POTATO FRIES
with GARLIC AND TRUFFLE OIL

With this recipe, we wanted to try a little something different with sweet potato fries. We love the mix of the sweetness of the sweet potato with the savory of the truffle oil and garlic. It's an unusual but delicious combination.

Preheat oven to 425°F.

In a large bowl, combine all the ingredients. Mix until the sweet potatoes are thoroughly coated. Place the sweet potatoes on a baking sheet lined with parchment paper in a single layer without touching each other. You might need to use more than one tray. Bake potatoes for 15 minutes, then flip them and bake until crispy at the edges, about 10 more minutes. Serve hot.

TIP You can use olive oil as a less expensive substitute for truffle oil.

MAKES 4 SERVINGS

2 medium sweet potatoes, cut into slices ¼ inch thick and the length of the potato

4 tablespoons truffle oil

1 tablespoon garlic powder

½ teaspoon sea salt

Freshly ground black pepper, to taste

HERBED POTATO SALAD

Classic (heavier, creamier) potato salad gets a lighter update in my mom's delicious recipe. The combination of horseradish mustard, apple cider vinegar, and thyme, along with other fresh seasonings, gives this potato salad a spicy kick and hearty flavor. And it tastes even better the second day. It's a great side dish for Peach BBQ Tempeh (page 183). And in terms of health benefits, the skin of red potatoes has three times more antioxidant power than white potatoes. Red potatoes are also a good source of vision-supporting and skin-nurturing vitamin A, bone-strengthening potassium, and colon-cleansing fiber.

3 pounds medium red potatoes, scrubbed well (not peeled)

2 tablespoons extra-virgin olive oil

1 large red onion, chopped

1 tablespoon horseradish mustard

3 tablespoons apple cider vinegar

2 teaspoons thyme

1 teaspoon sea salt, or to taste

1/8 teaspoon pepper, or to taste

1 cup finely chopped scallions

Place the potatoes in a large pot, cover with water, and bring to a boil. Then simmer, covered, over medium heat until tender and a fork can be inserted into the potatoes, 20 to 25 minutes.

In a large skillet, heat the oil over medium heat. Stir in the onions and sauté until translucent, 3 to 5 minutes. In a separate bowl, combine mustard, vinegar, thyme, salt, and pepper.

Drain potatoes and run cold water over them until just cool enough to handle. Peel the potatoes and cut them into cubes. Place the potatoes in a large bowl and add the seasonings mixture and onions. Toss gently and fold in the scallions. Taste and adjust the seasonings, as desired. Serve warm or at room temperature.

MAKES 8-10 SERVINGS

AGELESS ANTIOXIDANTS   BRAIN BOOSTER   HEALTH IS IN THE HUE   LONGEVITY LOVER
PROTEIN DREAM   SMOOTH SKIN   STRONG BONES   SUPER GREENS   VISION MISSION

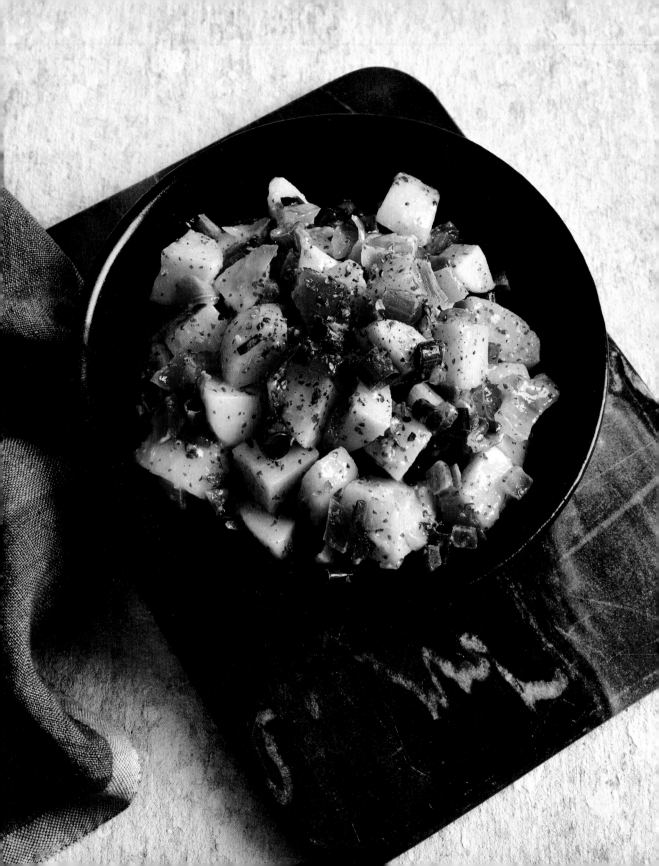

SPICED AND SAUTÉED
Sweet Potatoes

My mom loves sweet potatoes! She could eat them every day. So years ago she came up with a vegan version of the candied sweet potatoes she grew up with. They're light and buttery, with just a touch of added sweetness. They've become a family favorite and they make a perfect side dish for everyday meals or holiday feasts. We also love that sweet potatoes are so healthy. They're high in potassium, which helps protect bones and improve muscle strength, among other benefits.

3   medium sweet potatoes

1   tablespoon extra-virgin coconut oil

½   teaspoon ground cinnamon

⅛   teaspoon ground nutmeg

1   tablespoon maple syrup

½   tablespoon lemon juice (about ¼ lemon)

Preheat oven to 350°F.

Place the sweet potatoes in a baking pan and bake until cooked but still firm (not mushy), about 45 minutes. Let them cool down a bit so they're comfortable to the touch, then peel the potatoes and slice into ¼-inch-thick circles or chunks.

In a large skillet, heat the oil over low heat. Add the remaining ingredients. Stir until combined. Add the sweet potatoes and sauté for about 1 minute. Serve hot.

MAKES 4 SERVINGS

BLACK-EYED PEAS SALAD

This protein-packed recipe has a light, vibrant, and tangy dressing that pairs well with the earthy and nutty taste of black-eyed peas. The salad tastes even better the next day, when the seasonings have had more time to marinate. This dish is great on its own or as a topping for toasted pita chips (see recipe on page 112).

In a large bowl, toss together the black-eyed peas, tomato, corn, bell pepper, onion, garlic, and jalapeño. In a separate bowl, whisk together the lemon juice, vinegar, seasoning blend, and maple syrup (if using). Stir the juice mixture into the black-eyed peas mixture. Taste and adjust seasonings, as desired. Serve topped with avocado cubes.

MAKES 4-6 SERVINGS

- 2 (15-ounce) cans black-eyed peas, drained and rinsed
- 1 large tomato, diced
- 1 cup corn, fresh or cooked from frozen according to package instructions
- 1 red bell pepper, seeds removed, diced
- ½ medium red onion, diced
- 2 garlic cloves, finely chopped
- 1 jalapeño, seeded and finely chopped
- 2 tablespoons freshly squeezed lemon juice (about 1 lemon)
- 1 tablespoon coconut vinegar or red wine vinegar
- 2 teaspoons all-purpose dried herbs and vegetables seasoning blend
- 1 teaspoon maple syrup (optional)
- 1 avocado, pitted and cubed

CAJUN QUINOA
with OKRA AND TOMATO

Quinoa is my staple grain, so I love finding new ways to eat it. This recipe has a spicy Cajun mix of flavors that complement the mildness of quinoa nicely. And the added bonus: the okra stays nice and firm. So if you avoid okra because it can be soft and slimy, have no fear. This dish just might become your new okra staple. And not just for the flavor, but for the nutrients—okra is high in vitamin K and potassium, which help strengthen bones.

1 cup quinoa

1 tablespoon extra-virgin olive oil

½ medium yellow onion, thinly sliced

1 garlic clove, finely chopped

2 cups sliced okra

2 cups cherry tomatoes, cut in half

1½ teaspoons smoked paprika (or plain paprika)

½ teaspoon sea salt, or more to taste

Freshly ground black pepper, to taste

½ teaspoon dried oregano

1 teaspoon fresh thyme

Cayenne pepper, to taste

Put quinoa in a medium pot with 2 cups water and bring to a boil. Reduce the heat to low, cover, and simmer until tender and the liquid has been absorbed, 15 to 20 minutes. Remove from the heat and fluff with a fork.

In a large skillet, heat the oil over medium heat. Stir in the onions and garlic, and sauté until the onions are translucent, 3 to 5 minutes, stirring often. Add the okra and sauté until it starts to brown, about 5 minutes. Add the remaining ingredients and combine thoroughly. Sauté for 5 minutes. Gently stir in the quinoa and serve.

MAKES 4 SERVINGS

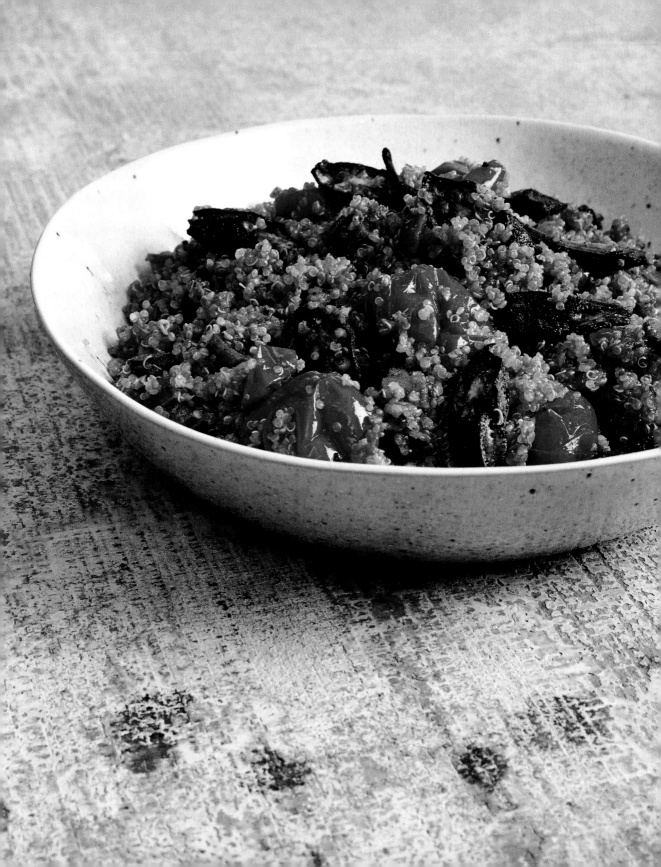

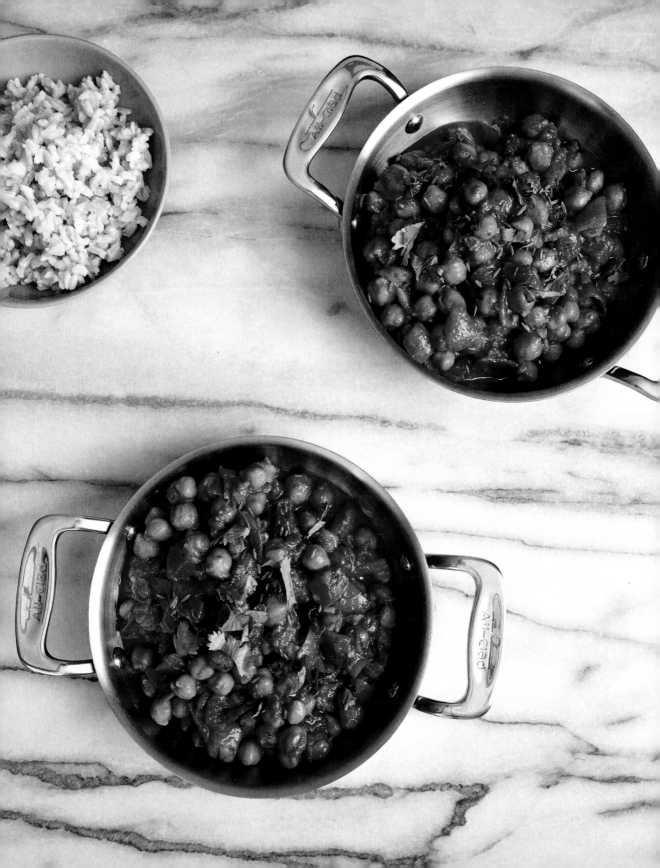

CHANA MASALA

This classic, spicy chickpea curry is a staple dish of India and has become one of the world's most popular foods. And it's one of my personal favorites, too. The spice blend that creates the curry's distinct flavor includes garam masala, cumin, turmeric, and coriander—all richly colored, aromatic spices that reflect their abundance of health-promoting and disease-fighting nutrients. This dish pairs well with Saffron Rice (page 131), Collards and Quinoa (page 165), and Roasted Curried Cauliflower (page 168).

In a soup pot, heat the oil over medium heat. Stir in the onions, garlic, and ginger, and sauté until the onions are translucent, 3 to 5 minutes. Add the paprika, coriander, ground cumin, turmeric, cumin seeds, and garam masala and sauté for 1 minute, stirring constantly. Add the tomatoes and 1 cup water. Stir the mixture, scraping the bottom of the pot to make sure the spices are not stuck to the bottom. Stir in the chickpeas, cayenne, and salt. Reduce the heat to low, cover, and simmer for 15 minutes, stirring occasionally. Just before serving, stir in lemon juice and top with cilantro.

MAKES 4 SERVINGS

1 tablespoon extra-virgin coconut oil

1 medium yellow onion, diced

1 garlic clove, finely chopped

1 tablespoon peeled and grated ginger

2 teaspoons paprika

1 teaspoon ground coriander

1 teaspoon ground cumin

1 teaspoon turmeric

1 teaspoon cumin seeds

1 teaspoon garam masala

2 medium tomatoes, chopped

3 cups precooked chickpeas, drained or 2 (15-ounce) cans or cartons

¼ teaspoon cayenne pepper, to taste

½ teaspoon sea salt

1 tablespoon freshly squeezed lemon juice (about ½ lemon)

½ cup chopped cilantro leaves

MAC AND CHEESE

This healthier vegan mac and cheese is deliciously flavored, perfectly seasoned, and firmly textured. And of course, it's cholesterol-free. The nutritional yeast, paprika, turmeric, and dried herbs seasonings also add distinct, disease-fighting antioxidants. And to make the dish even healthier, try adding 1 cup of finely chopped fresh spinach or broccoli florets for a boost of superfood vegetables.

2 cups small whole-grain elbow noodles

1¼ cups plain, unsweetened soy or almond milk

½ cup safflower, grapeseed, or other nonflavored oil

½ cup nutritional yeast

5 garlic cloves

1 teaspoon all-purpose dried herbs and vegetables seasoning blend

¼ teaspoon paprika

¼ teaspoon black pepper

⅛ teaspoon sea salt

⅛ teaspoon turmeric

⅛ teaspoon cayenne pepper

Preheat oven to 350°F.

Cook noodles al dente, according to package instructions, and set aside. In a blender, add the remaining ingredients. Blend on low until smooth and creamy. Taste and adjust seasonings, as desired. In a large bowl, combine the milk mixture and noodles. Place in a 13 x 9-inch baking dish. Bake, uncovered, for 40 to 50 minutes, or until the top of the mac and cheese is golden brown and the edges start to crisp. Serve hot.

TIPS For individual mac-n-cheese cups, divide scoops of the mixture among the cups of a 12-tin muffin tin, rather than a baking dish.

This mac and cheese has a thick cheese sauce. If you prefer a thinner sauce, add ¼ to ½ cup more milk.

MAKES 6-8 SERVINGS

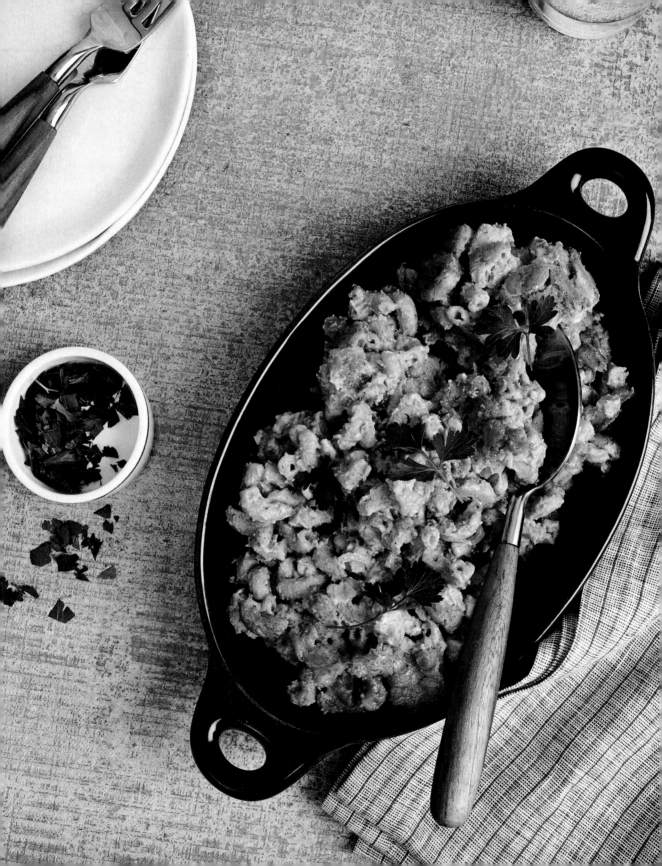

BLACK BEAN SOUP
with AVOCADO AND CASHEW SOUR CREAM

If you're craving a warming, comforting soup that tastes good to your soul, this is it. Black beans are higher in antioxidants than most beans, which means they're most effective against cell-damaging free radicals that can result in premature aging. Their high fiber content also lowers the risk of chronic diseases and increases longevity.

1 tablespoon extra-virgin olive oil

1 large carrot, peeled and sliced into thin rounds

½ red onion, coarsely chopped

4 garlic cloves, finely chopped

3 cups precooked black beans or 2 (15-ounce) cans or cartons

2 tablespoons low-sodium tamari

2 tablespoons hot salsa (see Tip)

7 cherry tomatoes, halved

2 tablespoons nutritional yeast

½ teaspoon cayenne pepper

1 avocado, pitted and cut into chunks

3 tablespoons finely chopped fresh cilantro

Cashew Sour Cream (page 102)

In a large skillet, heat the oil over medium heat. Stir in the carrots, onions, and garlic and sauté until the onions are translucent, 3 to 5 minutes. In a large pot, bring 2 cups water to a simmer over low heat. Add the beans, carrots, onions, and garlic, plus the tamari, salsa, tomatoes, nutritional yeast, and cayenne pepper. Simmer over low heat, covered, for about 10 minutes. Serve hot, topped with avocado chunks, cilantro, and a dollop of Cashew Sour Cream. This soup freezes well in airtight containers, so it can be made in large batches and stored for lunch and dinner during the week.

TIP To make homemade salsa, see page 102.

MAKES 4 SERVINGS

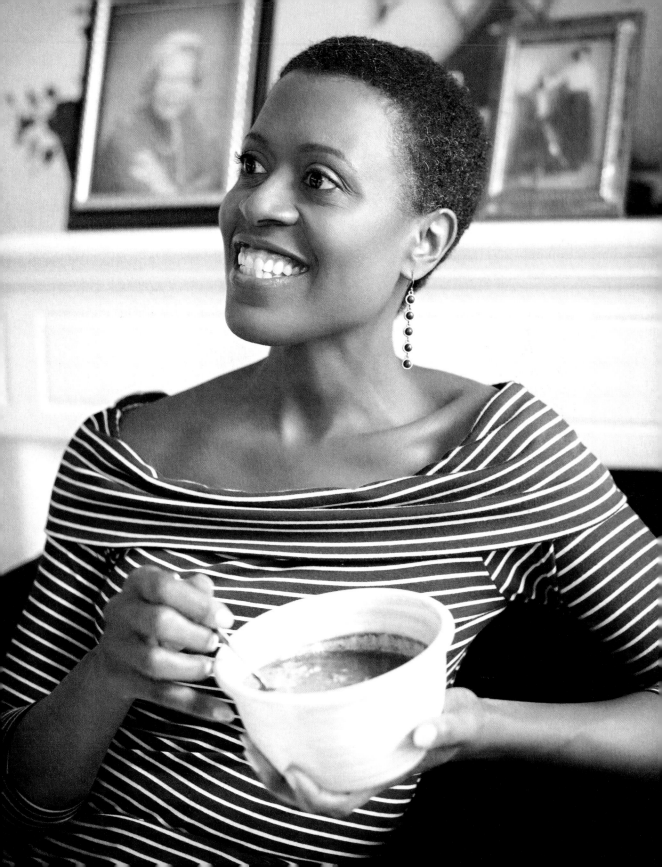

Vegetables

Because vegetables are such an integral part of what we eat every day, we know variety is essential to keep them interesting, nutritious, and delicious. So the dishes in this chapter incorporate more than twenty types of colorful vegetables. And the preparation methods range from raw to roasted. Some highlights include Arugula Salad with Walnuts and Caesar Dressing (you'll want to pour the dressing on everything!); charred and tangy Balsamic Brussels Sprouts; and light and flavorful String Beans with Shiitake Mushrooms and Almonds.

Arugula Salad with Walnuts and Caesar Dressing

Sesame Spiced Edamame

Swiss Chard Sauté with Walnuts

Citrusy Dandelion Greens Salad

String Beans with Shiitake Mushrooms and Almonds

Roasted Corn on the Cob with Spicy Rub

Roasted Root Vegetables

Balsamic Brussels Sprouts

All Hail the Kale Salad Remix

Spicy Beet Greens

Roasted Beet Slices with Rosemary

Collards and Quinoa

Braised Sesame Kale

Rainbow Slaw

Roasted Curried Cauliflower

ARUGULA SALAD
with WALNUTS AND CAESAR DRESSING

The base of this leafy green salad is arugula, a good source of lutein and zeaxanthin, which help promote eye health and protect against macular degeneration. The garlicky Caesar dressing perfectly balances the arugula's strong, distinct flavor. I toss the salad with protein-rich Crunchy Roasted Chickpeas (page 106) to round out the meal. The Caesar dressing also pairs wonderfully well with All Hail the Kale Salad Remix (page 160) and Rainbow Slaw (page 167). And finally, the optional edible flowers add a dose of colorful nutrients as a garnish. The rich hues reflect an abundance of antioxidants that can help ward off diseases from heart disease to cancer.

CAESAR DRESSING

- 2 tablespoons whole-grain mustard
- 2 tablespoons nutritional yeast
- 2 tablespoons almond meal
- ¼ teaspoon finely chopped garlic
- 2 tablespoons freshly squeezed lemon juice (about 1 lemon)
- 1 teaspoon low-sodium tamari
- 1 tablespoon extra-virgin olive oil
- ½ teaspoon sea salt
  Freshly ground black pepper, to taste
  Cayenne pepper, to taste

SALAD

- 4 cups arugula
- 1 cup red grapes, halved
- ½ cup raw walnuts
- 20 edible flowers, such as violas (optional)

In a blender, combine all the dressing ingredients with ¼ cup water. Blend until smooth and creamy. Place arugula, grapes, and walnuts in a large bowl and toss with dressing. Taste and adjust salt and pepper, as desired. If using, add edible flowers before serving.

TIP The optional edible flowers can be found at farmers' markets, grocery stores, and online or you can grow your own.

MAKES 4 SERVINGS

AGELESS ANTIOXIDANTS   BRAIN BOOSTER   HEALTH IS IN THE HUE   LONGEVITY LOVER
PROTEIN DREAM   SMOOTH SKIN   STRONG BONES   SUPER GREENS   VISION MISSION

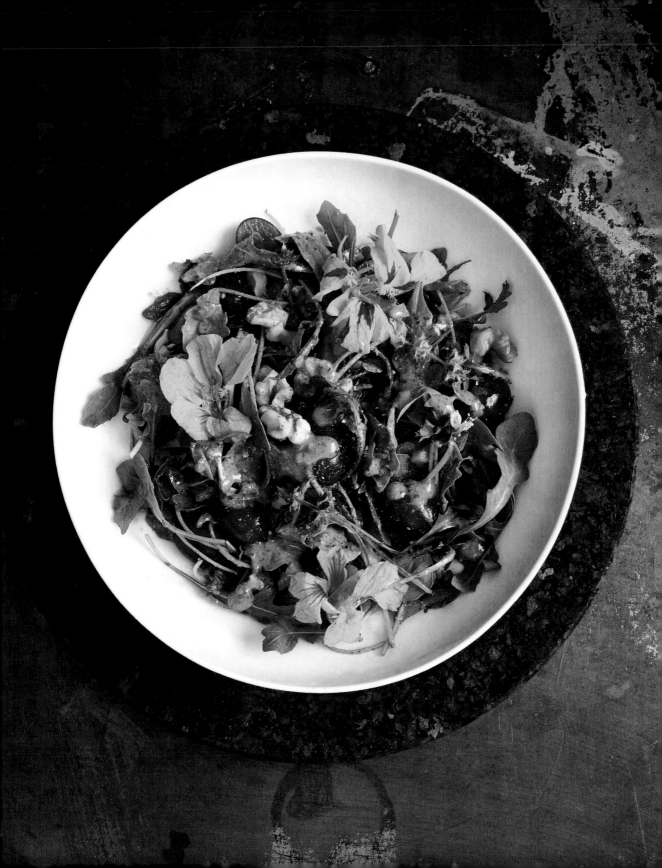

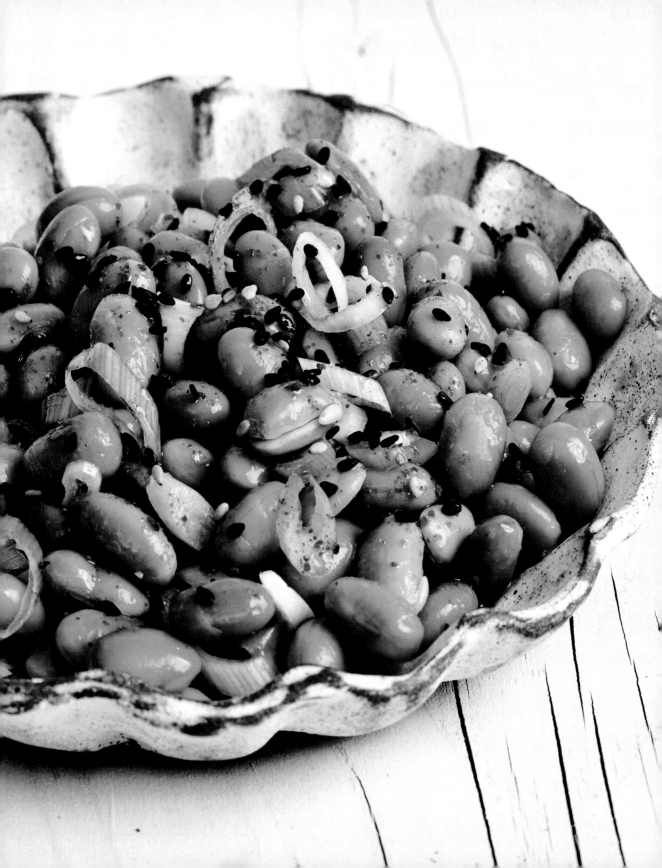

SESAME SPICED EDAMAME

Edamame is a young soybean high in protein, fiber, calcium, and iron—all key nutrients for better health and longevity. You'll love the crunchy yet soft and smooth consistency of the edamame in this recipe, which is coated with a spicy sesame oil dressing and sprinkled with black sesame seeds, which help protect bone health. It tastes great tossed with whole-grain pasta noodles, like our Buckwheat Soba Bowl recipe (page 182) or with our Citrusy Dandelion Greens Salad (page 153).

In a large bowl, combine all the ingredients. Mix thoroughly and serve at room temperature.

MAKES 4 SERVINGS

2 cups edamame, cooked according to package directions

1 tablespoon toasted sesame oil

1 tablespoon sesame seeds (black, brown, or mixed)

1 teaspoon sea salt

2 tablespoons finely chopped scallions

Cayenne pepper, to taste

Swiss Chard Sauté
with WALNUTS

The sweet and savory combination of currants and Swiss chard, combined with the toasty flavor of baked walnuts, make this dish a standout. Swiss chard is also a standout for being high in the antioxidants lutein and zeaxanthin, which are two of your best protectors against macular degeneration as you get older. This dish pairs well with Spiced and Sautéed Sweet Potatoes (page 136) and Peach BBQ Tempeh (page 183).

⅓ cup raw walnuts, roughly chopped

1 bunch Swiss chard

¼ cup currants

1 tablespoon extra-virgin olive oil

¼ teaspoon sea salt or more, to taste

Freshly ground black pepper, to taste

Preheat oven to 350°F.

Line a baking sheet with parchment paper. Place walnuts on the lined sheet in a single layer and bake until golden brown, about 8 minutes. Place chard and 3 tablespoons water in a large pot. Turn heat to medium, cover, and simmer about 5 minutes, stirring often, until greens are wilted. Remove from heat and stir in the currants, walnuts, oil, salt, and pepper. Mix until thoroughly combined. Serve hot.

MAKES 4 SERVINGS

CITRUSY
DANDELION GREENS SALAD

You might be surprised at how rich, creamy, and delicious this salad is. The bitterness that dandelion greens are known for is mellowed by the garlicky lemon dressing, avocado, and pine nuts. It might just become one of your favorite salads, as it is for me. That's no surprise—dandelion greens are probably my favorite greens. They're high in the antioxidants lutein and zeaxanthin, which help promote eye health and protect against macular degeneration, and in vitamin K, which helps maintain bone health. This salad pairs well with Tempeh Panini (page 172) and Curried Chickpeas in Warm Pita Pocket (page 197).

Preheat oven to 375°F.

Place the garlic cloves in a small bowl and toss with ½ teaspoon of the oil. Place on a baking sheet and bake until soft, about 15 minutes. Let cool until easy to touch, about 5 minutes, and remove the skins.

Place dandelion greens, pine nuts, and avocado slices in a bowl and gently toss. In a blender, combine the roasted garlic, remaining oil, 1 tablespoon water, lemon juice, salt, and pepper. Blend until smooth. Pour the lemon dressing over the dandelion greens salad and gently toss. Add more salt and pepper, if needed. Serve immediately.

MAKES 4 SERVINGS

3 unpeeled garlic cloves

2 tablespoons plus ½ teaspoon extra-virgin olive oil

1 bunch dandelion greens, stems removed and leaves chopped into 2-inch pieces

¼ cup pine nuts

1 avocado, pitted and sliced

3 tablespoons freshly squeezed lemon juice (about 1 lemon)

½ teaspoon sea salt
   Freshly ground black pepper, to taste

STRING BEANS
with SHIITAKE MUSHROOMS AND ALMONDS

These quick and easy green beans and immune-boosting shiitake mushrooms are oven-broiled (instead of stir-fried or sautéed) for a lovely, smoky flavor. They're finished with crunchy raw almonds and a kick of hot sauce. This dish pairs well with Peach BBQ Tempeh (page 183), Herbed Potato Salad (page 134), and Mac and Cheese (page 142).

1 pound string beans

2 cups shiitake mushrooms, thinly sliced

¼ medium white onion, very finely chopped (about 2 tablespoons)

1 tablespoon extra-virgin olive oil

1 teaspoon sea salt

Freshly ground black pepper, to taste

¼ cup raw almonds, roughly chopped

Hot sauce

Preheat oven to broil.

After washing the string beans and mushrooms, make sure to pat them dry thoroughly so they don't steam in the broiler. In a large bowl, combine the string beans, mushrooms, onion, oil, salt, and pepper. Mix thoroughly. Place the mixture on a baking sheet lined with parchment paper that is large enough to hold the ingredients in a single layer. Cook under the broiler until browned, 5 to 8 minutes, checking often to make sure they don't burn. Top with almonds and serve with hot sauce.

MAKES 4 SERVINGS

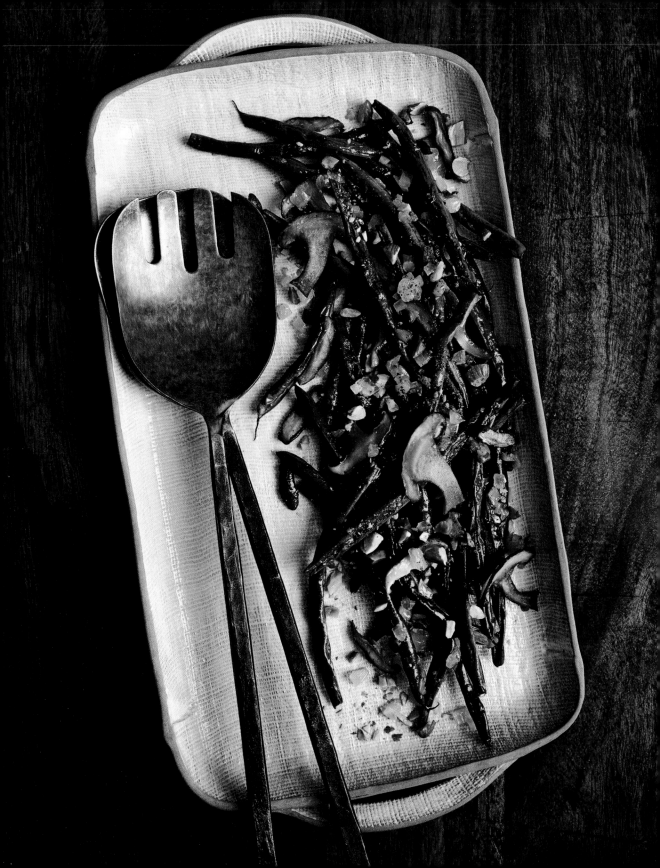

ROASTED CORN ON THE COB
with SPICY RUB

Fresh, buttery, and spicy, this oven-roasted corn on the cob is a must-have for your summertime cook-outs. The antioxidants in corn also help to improve vision and help skin stay smooth. This Roasted Corn on the Cob goes great with Colorful Kebab (page 179) and Peach BBQ Tempeh (page 183).

4 ears corn, husks removed
2 tablespoons extra-virgin coconut oil
1 tablespoon chili powder
2 tablespoons nutritional yeast
½ teaspoon sea salt

Preheat oven to 400°F.

Place corn in a 13 x 9-inch baking pan and rub oil on corn until thoroughly coated. Combine the chili powder, nutritional yeast, and salt in a bowl. Sprinkle half of the mixture on one side of the corn. Cover the pan with foil and roast for about 15 minutes. Turn the corn over, sprinkle it with the remaining spice mixture, cover, and roast for 10 more minutes. Serve hot.

MAKES 4 SERVINGS

ROASTED ROOT VEGETABLES

This is healthy, warming, comfort food at its best. Roasting root vegetables releases their naturally sweet flavor. And seasonings like olive oil, rosemary, and oregano give them just the right amount of savory flavor to complement the sweet. Rosemary and carrots also add ageless antioxidants to the mix that improve brain function, memory, and vision. For this dish, you can use any colorful combination of root vegetables you'd like. They pair well with Three-Bean Chili (page 204) and Crispy Tofu Bites (page 111).

Preheat oven to 350°F.

In a large bowl, add all the vegetables except red beets, but if you're using gold ones, they're fine to add now. Drizzle the vegetables with the oil and make sure they're evenly coated. Add seasonings to the vegetables and mix well. Gently fold in the red beets (your goal here is to minimize staining the other vegetables red). Place all vegetables, except onions, on a baking sheet lined with parchment paper. Cook for 15 minutes, then turn over the vegetables and add in the onions. Cover loosely with foil and cook for 10 more minutes. Serve hot.

MAKES 6-8 SERVINGS

8 small multicolored carrots, sliced on an angle

5 Japanese sweet potatoes, sliced into ½-inch wedges

4 red or golden beets, sliced into ½-inch wedges

2 large red onions, sliced into rounds

2 small red radishes, sliced into rounds

3 tablespoons extra-virgin olive oil

1 teaspoon oregano

1 teaspoon basil

1 teaspoon rosemary

1 teaspoon red pepper flakes

¼ teaspoon sea salt, or to taste

Black pepper to taste

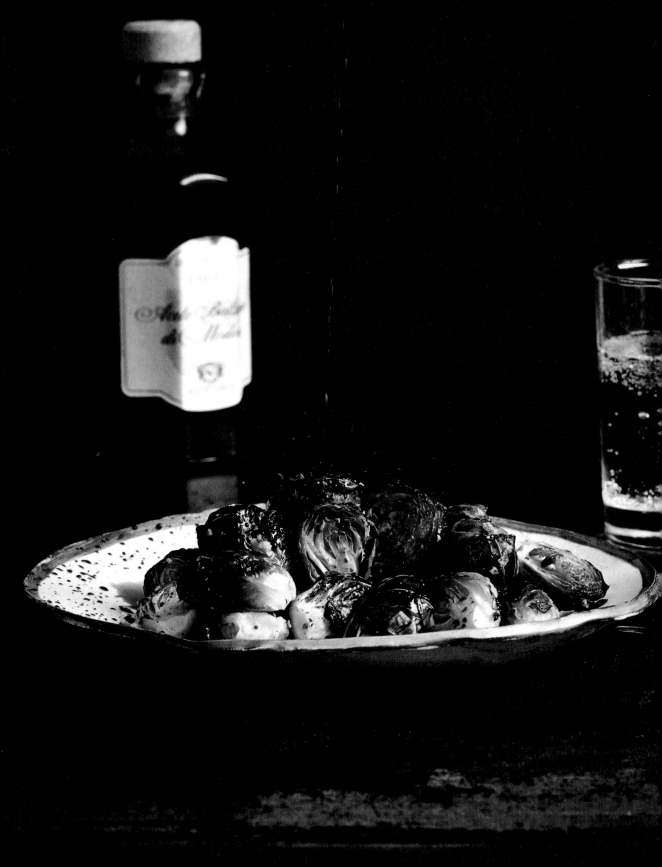

BALSAMIC BRUSSELS SPROUTS

Pop these roasted and seasoned Brussels sprouts in your mouth and taste the layers of flavor unleashed: fresh, charred, sweet, tangy, savory, and spicy. Simple and easy to prepare, these Brussels sprouts make a healthy and delectable side dish or snack. As a heart-healthy and cancer-fighting cruciferous vegetable, Brussels sprouts are nutrition powerhouses for health and longevity. This dish goes well with Mac and Cheese (page 142) and Savory Vegetable Quiche (page 200).

Preheat oven to 400°F.

In a large bowl, combine the Brussels sprouts, oil, garlic, salt, and pepper, making sure they're evenly coated. Place Brussels sprouts on a baking sheet lined with parchment paper. Roast until crisp and golden brown on the outside and tender on the inside, 20 to 30 minutes. Shake the pan about every 10 minutes to be sure they're evenly roasted. Remove from the oven, immediately drizzle with vinegar, and toss until evenly coated. Sprinkle with additional salt and pepper, if needed. Serve hot.

MAKES 4 SERVINGS

1 pound Brussels sprouts, cut in half, ends trimmed and yellow leaves removed

3 tablespoons extra-virgin olive oil

3 garlic cloves, finely chopped

½ teaspoon sea salt

Freshly ground black pepper, to taste

2 tablespoons balsamic vinegar

All Hail the Kale
SALAD REMIX

This is the most popular recipe from my first book, *By Any Greens Necessary*, and one that I personally make a few times a week. It's absolutely delish! I've updated it with freshly squeezed lemon juice for a citrusy twist, along with my latest favorite toppings: pecans, grated carrots, avocados, and cherry tomatoes. The beauty of this salad is that it has the perfect dressing of olive oil, tamari, and nutritional yeast, so it'll always taste great with whatever toppings you choose. And with bone-strengthening and vision-protecting kale as its foundation, this salad is also super nutritious. It goes great with Crunchy Roasted Chickpeas (page 106), Tempeh Panini (page 172), and Savory Vegetable Quiche (page 200).

2–3 bunches curly kale, coarsely chopped

3 tablespoons extra-virgin olive oil

2 tablespoons low-sodium tamari

1 tablespoon freshly squeezed lemon juice (about ½ lemon)

2 tablespoons nutritional yeast

¼ teaspoon cayenne pepper

1 medium red onion, chopped

5 garlic cloves, peeled and chopped

½ cup grated carrot (about 1 medium carrot)

1 cup whole pecans

1 avocado, pitted and cubed

1 cup cherry tomatoes, halved

Place the kale in a large bowl and drizzle on the oil, tamari, and lemon juice. Toss to make sure all the leaves are coated. Sprinkle on nutritional yeast and cayenne pepper and toss again to make sure all the leaves are coated. Add onion, garlic, carrot, and pecans and toss well. Let marinate at room temperature for about 15 minutes so the kale leaves can wilt a little. Serve topped with avocado and tomatoes.

MAKES 6-8 SERVINGS

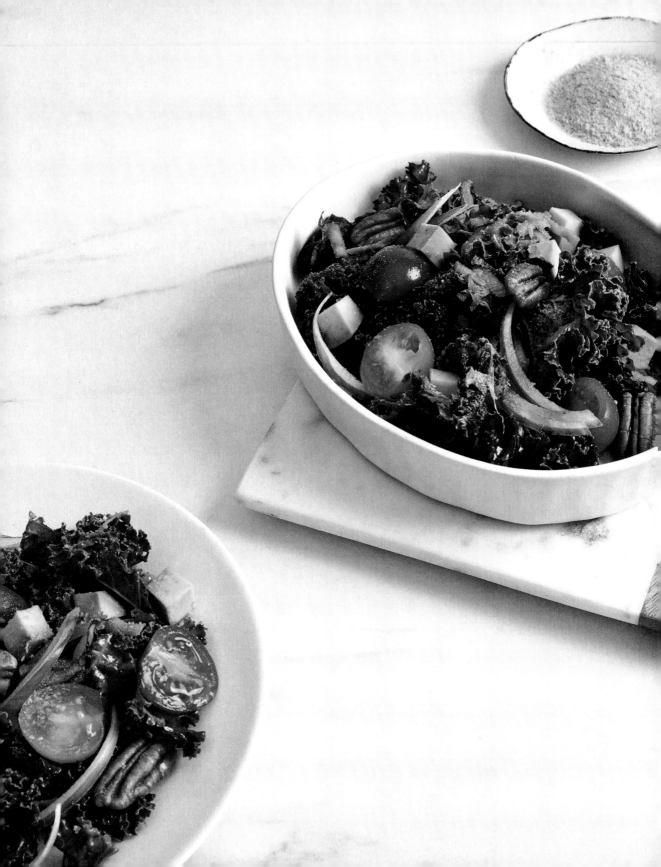

SPICY BEET GREENS

These tender, iron-rich, and heart-healthy leaves are divine when lightly sautéed with just a few simple seasonings to enhance the subtle, aromatic flavor of the greens and they take just a few minutes to prepare. They're also delicious raw when added to a salad or tossed into a morning smoothie. This dish goes well with Saffron Rice (page 131) and Chana Masala (page 141).

1 tablespoon sesame oil

4 garlic cloves, finely chopped

2 bunches beet greens

2 tablespoons coconut aminos or low-sodium tamari

½ teaspoon red pepper flakes

In a large skillet, heat the oil over medium heat. Stir in the garlic and sauté until translucent, 3 to 5 minutes. Stir in the greens, coconut aminos, and pepper flakes and sauté for 1 to 2 more minutes. Beet greens wilt quickly, so be careful not to overcook them. Serve hot.

MAKES 4 SERVINGS

ROASTED BEET SLICES
with ROSEMARY

The roasted beets in this dish are slightly crispy on the outside and tender on the inside, infused with the aromatic flavor of fresh rosemary. They taste great on their own or sliced and added to salads, like Arugula Salad with Walnuts and Caesar Dressing (page 148) and All Hail the Kale Salad Remix (page 160). Rosemary is an antioxidant-rich herb that helps improve memory and brain functioning.

Preheat oven to 450°F.

Line a baking sheet with parchment paper and set aside. Place beets in a bowl, coat with oil and add the remaining ingredients. Toss to evenly distribute the seasonings. Place beets in a single layer on the lined baking sheet. Bake until the edges of the beets are brown and the centers are tender, 30 to 40 minutes, checking often to make sure they don't burn. Serve hot or at room temperature.

MAKES 4-6 SERVINGS

3 medium unpeeled beets in different colors, cut into ⅛-inch slices

1 tablespoon extra-virgin olive oil

2 shallots, finely chopped

1½ tablespoons finely chopped rosemary

1 teaspoon sea salt
    Freshly ground black pepper, to taste

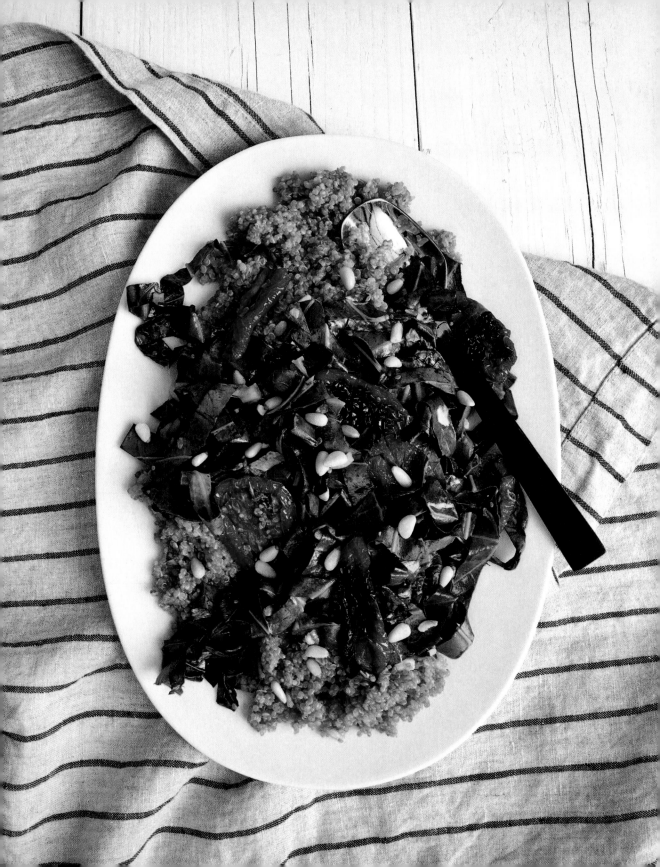

COLLARDS AND QUINOA

This is another dish I love to eat about once a week. The tart taste of collards and sun-dried tomatoes blends so wonderfully with the curry flavor and smooth texture of the quinoa. It's simple, comforting, and satisfying. Collards are also exceptionally high in vitamin K, helping to promote bone strength and increase bone density. This dish pairs well with Three-Bean Chili (page 204), Mac and Cheese (page 142), and Southern-Style Cornbread (page 128).

QUINOA Place the quinoa and 2 cups water in a medium pot and bring to a boil. Reduce the heat to low, add the seasonings, cover, and simmer for 20 minutes or until the water is completely absorbed.

COLLARDS In a large skillet, heat the oil over medium heat. Stir in the onions and garlic, and sauté until the onions are translucent, 3 to 5 minutes. Stir in the collards and sauté for 2 to 3 more minutes or until the collards just start to wilt. Add the tomatoes, pine nuts, and seasonings and sauté for 2 more minutes. The collards should be slightly wilted and still bright green. Top the quinoa with the collards and serve immediately.

MAKES 4-5 SERVINGS

QUINOA
- 1 cup quinoa
- 1 teaspoon turmeric or curry powder
  Pinch sea salt

COLLARDS
- 1 tablespoon extra-virgin olive oil
- ¼ medium red onion, diced
- 4 garlic cloves, finely chopped
- 1 bunch collard greens, bottom stems removed, cut into thin strips
- ¼ cup halved sun-dried tomatoes (about 8 to 10 tomatoes)
- ¼ cup raw pine nuts
- 2 tablespoons nutritional yeast
- 1 tablespoon low-sodium tamari
- ¼ teaspoon cayenne pepper or dash hot sauce, to taste

Braised Sesame Kale

During the colder winter months or around the holidays, these braised greens hit the spot, especially paired with Mac and Cheese (page 142) and Crispy Tofu Bites (page 111).

1 tablespoon extra-virgin olive oil

¼ medium red onion, diced

1 large bunch kale, stems removed and coarsely chopped

¼ cup low-sodium vegetable stock

¼ teaspoon sea salt, or to taste

Black pepper, to taste

½ teaspoon raw sesame seeds

In a large skillet, heat the oil over medium heat. Stir in the onions and sauté until translucent, 3 to 5 minutes. Stir in the kale and sauté for 2 to 3 minutes or until just wilted. Add remaining ingredients, except the sesame seeds, and cook for 2 to 3 more minutes. Using a slotted spoon to drain the liquid, place the kale on a plate, sprinkle sesame seeds on top, and serve immediately.

MAKES 4 SERVINGS

AGELESS ANTIOXIDANTS   BRAIN BOOSTER   HEALTH IS IN THE HUE   LONGEVITY LOVER
PROTEIN DREAM   SMOOTH SKIN   STRONG BONES   SUPER GREENS   VISION MISSION

Rainbow Slaw

This vibrant, colorful salad tastes just as good as it looks. The more colors the better, because each color signifies particular phytonutrients that can help prevent and reverse chronic diseases and help you live a longer, healthier life. It's the perfect Health Is in the Hue dish. This dish goes well with Black-Eyed Peas Salad (page 137), Herbed Potato Salad (page 134), and Peach BBQ Tempeh (page 183).

In a large bowl, combine all the ingredients, except the avocados, making sure the vegetables are evenly coated with the dressing. Fold in the avocados and serve.

MAKES 4 SERVINGS

2 cups shredded purple cabbage (about one small head of cabbage)

1 cup corn, fresh or cooked from frozen according to package instructions

1 large carrot, shredded

1½ cups precooked black beans or 1 (15-ounce) can or carton

½ cup cherry tomatoes, halved

½ small red onion, chopped

3 garlic cloves, chopped
Caesar Dressing (page 148)

2 avocados, pitted and cubed

ROASTED CURRIED CAULIFLOWER

The combination of curry spices along with oven-roasting makes this cauliflower dish come alive. It's delicious and nutrient-rich—cauliflower is especially high in vitamin C, which supports healthy skin and strong bones. This dish pairs well with Chana Masala (page 141).

1 small head cauliflower cut into florets

1 tablespoon extra-virgin olive oil

½ teaspoon sea salt

Freshly ground black pepper, to taste

½ teaspoon ground turmeric

½ teaspoon smoked paprika

½ teaspoon whole cumin seeds

¼ teaspoon cayenne pepper

Hot sauce

Preheat oven to 450°F.

In a large bowl, add cauliflower and coat with oil, salt, pepper, turmeric, paprika, cumin seeds, and cayenne. Place cauliflower on a baking sheet lined with parchment paper, place in oven, and roast until golden brown, 7 to 10 minutes. Serve hot with toothpicks, with hot sauce on the side.

MAKES 4-6 SERVINGS

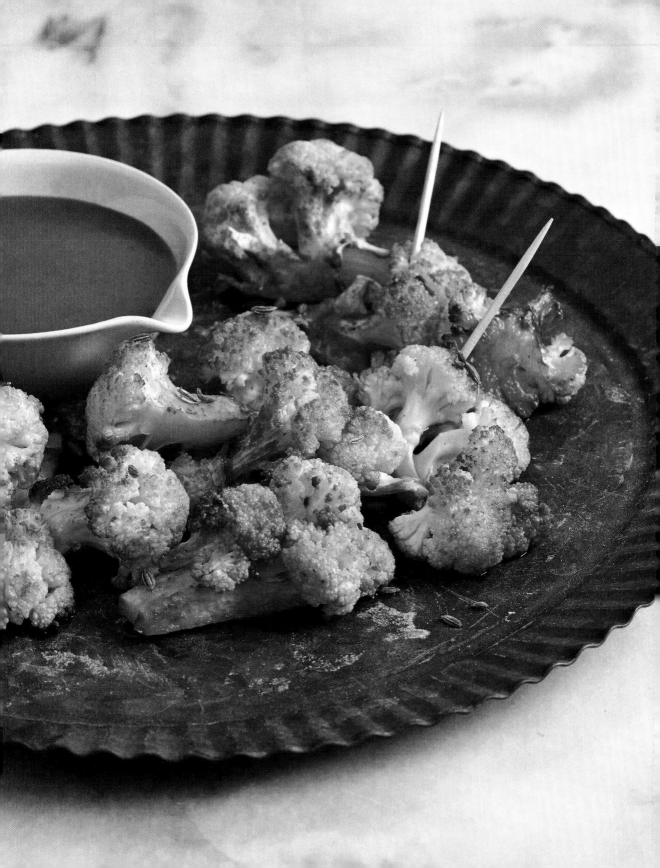

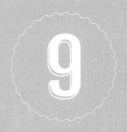

Entrées

For this chapter, we strolled down memory lane to bring you some of our favorite main dishes over the years, but with a new twist, including Savory Vegetable Quiche; Lasagna with Mushrooms, Eggplant, and Zucchini; Vegetable Pot Pie; and Stuffed Orange and Red Bell Peppers. And when time allows for more involved preparation, we think you'll love the Purple Cabbage Bowl and Ethiopian Platter—they're worth every minute.

Tempeh Panini

Purple Cabbage Bowl

Pinto Bean Wrap

Colorful Kebab

Pad Thai

Buckwheat Soba Bowl

Peach BBQ Tempeh

Spicy Basil Eggplant with Dates, Cashews, and Brown Rice

Stuffed Orange and Red Bell Peppers

Lasagna with Mushrooms, Eggplant, and Zucchini

Enchiladas

Basil Mushroom Pizza

Vegetable Stir-Fry with Black Rice and Almond Butter Sauce

Roasted Sweet Potato and Black Bean Bowl with Lime Cilantro Vinaigrette

Curried Chickpeas in Warm Pita Pocket

Vegetable Pot Pie

Savory Vegetable Quiche

Ethiopian Platter

Three-Bean Chili

TEMPEH PANINI

This panini is an updated twist on the BLT sandwich I loved as a child, this time made with hearty tempeh and a tangy pesto made with arugula, sun-dried tomatoes, and pine nuts for a rich, creamy taste. The panini is packed with protein from the tempeh and pine nuts, with heart-healthy and cancer-fighting antioxidants from the arugula greens, and cholesterol-lowering healthy fats from the avocado.

ARUGULA PESTO

- 2 cups arugula
- ½ cup dry sun-dried tomatoes, soaked in hot water for 20 minutes and drained
- 2 tablespoons extra-virgin olive oil
- 2 tablespoons pine nuts
- 2 tablespoons nutritional yeast
- 1 garlic clove, chopped
- ¼ teaspoon sea salt

TEMPEH

- 1 (8-ounce) package plain tempeh
- 1 tablespoon extra-virgin olive oil
- 1 tablespoon coconut aminos or low-sodium tamari
- 1 tablespoon balsamic vinegar
  Freshly ground black pepper, to taste

SANDWICH

- 8 (¼-inch) thick slices whole-grain bread
- 1 avocado, pitted and thinly sliced
- 1 large tomato, thinly sliced
- ½ teaspoon extra-virgin olive oil

Preheat oven to 375°F.

Line a baking sheet with parchment paper and set aside.

PESTO In a food processor, combine the pesto ingredients and process for 30 seconds.

TEMPEH Cut tempeh into ⅛-inch-thick strips. Place the strips in a bowl and gently coat with the oil, coconut aminos, vinegar, and pepper. Place on the lined baking sheet and bake until golden brown, about 10 minutes, flip and bake until the other side is golden brown, about 5 more minutes.

SANDWICH Heat a panini press or large, heavy-bottom skillet over medium heat.

Assemble sandwiches by evenly spreading the pesto on the eight slices of bread. Place the avocado and tomato slices on top of the pesto. Place the tempeh on top of the pesto on four of the slices and then cover the tempeh with the remaining four slices of bread.

Lightly coat press or pan with oil and place sandwiches in the pan. Cook until golden brown, about 5 minutes, then flip and cook for 5 more minutes. If you do not have a panini press, weigh the sandwiches down with a heavy pot or skillet. Serve warm or at room temperature.

MAKES 4 SERVINGS

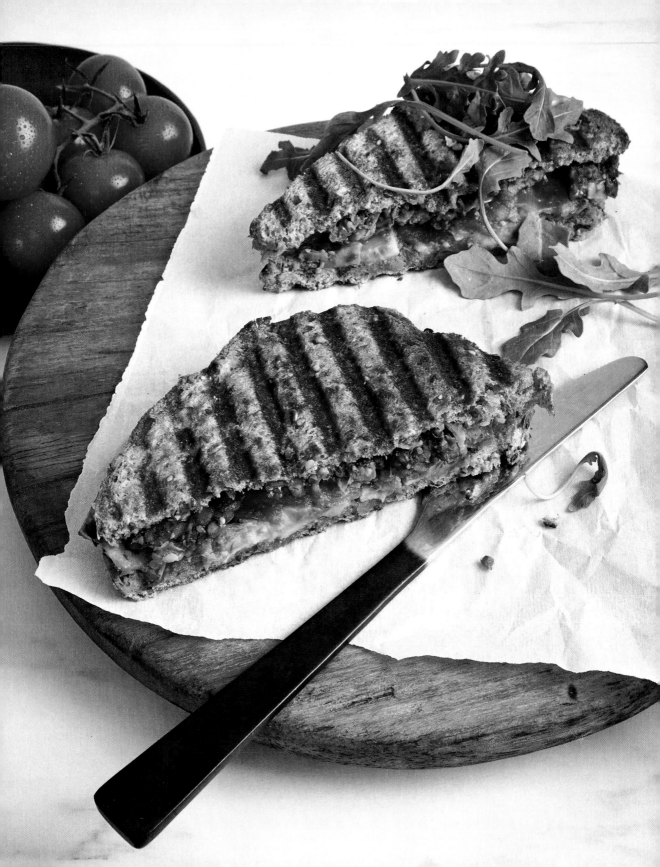

PURPLE CABBAGE BOWL

This pretty, hearty dish is a perfect example of Health Is in the Hue, with colorful foods that reflect their abundance of ageless antioxidants. There's vision-improving carrots, protein-packed tempeh, potassium-rich cabbage, immune-boosting beets, and more. Although there are multiple steps in this recipe, the delicious results make it all worthwhile.

TEMPEH

- 2 tablespoons white vinegar
- 1 tablespoon extra-virgin olive oil
- 1 tablespoon coconut aminos or low-sodium tamari
- 1 tablespoon balsamic vinegar
- 2 teaspoons whole-grain mustard
- 1 garlic clove, very finely chopped
- ½ teaspoon sea salt
- 1 (8-ounce) package plain tempeh

SAUCE

- ½ cup cashew butter
- ¼ cup coconut milk (light)
- 2 tablespoons rice vinegar
- 2 tablespoons freshly squeezed lime juice (about 1 lime)
- 1 tablespoon coconut aminos or low-sodium tamari
- 1 teaspoon toasted sesame oil
- 1 jalapeño
- ½ teaspoon peeled and grated ginger
- ½ teaspoon sea salt

SLAW

- 1 head red cabbage, 4 outer leaves carefully peeled away to use as bowls
- 2 cups thinly sliced red cabbage (from the same head mentioned above)
- ½ small napa cabbage, thinly sliced (about 2 cups)
- 1 medium carrot, spiral cut or shredded (about 1 cup)
- ½ medium beet, spiral cut or shredded (about 1 cup)
- ¼ cup chopped cilantro
- ¼ cup chopped raw cashews or cashew pieces
- 1 medium spring onion, thinly sliced, white part only (about 2 tablespoons)

RECIPE CONTINUED ON PAGE 176

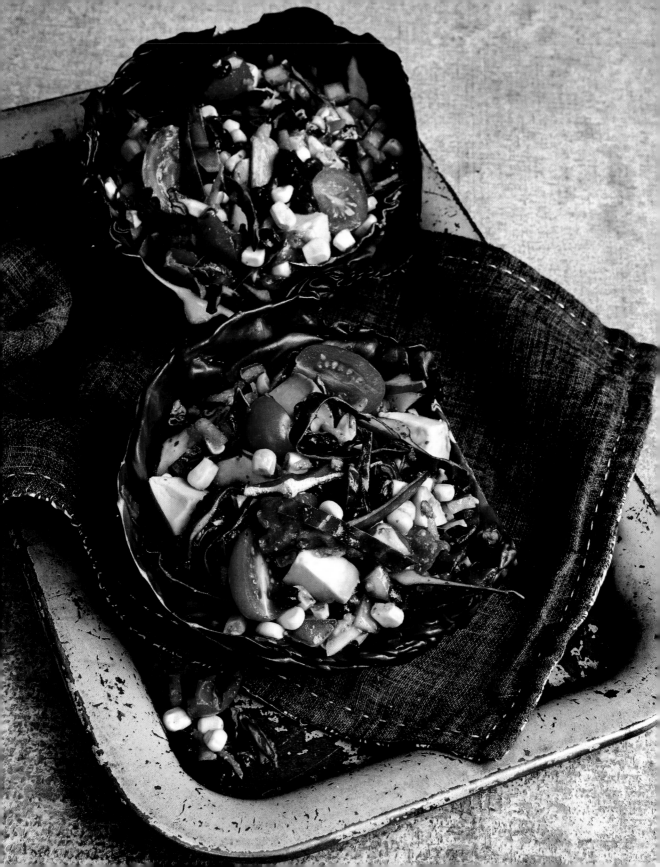

RECIPE CONTINUED FROM PAGE 174

TEMPEH Preheat oven to 375°F.

In a bowl, combine the vinegar, oil, coconut aminos, balsamic, mustard, garlic, and salt and mix thoroughly. Cut the tempeh into ¼-inch-thick strips and place in a 9 x 9-inch ovenproof dish that will hold all the strips in a single layer. Pour the vinegar mixture over the tempeh and let sit for 10 minutes, then flip the tempeh and let sit for 10 more minutes, so both sides get coated with the marinade. Place tempeh in the oven and bake for 10 minutes, then flip and bake for 10 more minutes, until browned on both sides. Chop the tempeh into small bite-sized pieces.

SAUCE In a blender, combine the sauce ingredients and blend until smooth.

SLAW In a large bowl, combine the tempeh, sliced red cabbage, napa cabbage, carrot, beet, cilantro, cashews, and spring onions. Add the sauce and mix until evenly coated. Divide the mixture between the 4 cabbage leaves.

MAKES 4 SERVINGS

PINTO BEAN WRAP

Besides being super nutritious and simple to make, one of the best things about bean wraps is their versatility. This recipe calls for pinto beans, but any beans would be delicious. Wraps are a great way to get a variety of protein-packed and fiber-filled beans onto your plate throughout the week.

BEANS In a food processor, combine the garlic, basil, oil, and vinegar until smooth. Add the beans, cayenne, salt, and pepper. Pulse on and off about five times for 5 seconds each, until the mixture is thoroughly combined, but there are still some pieces left about half the size of a pea. Taste and adjust seasonings, as desired.

ASSEMBLE Lay the wraps on a flat surface. Spread one-quarter of the bean mixture on each of the wraps to cover them. Stack the avocado, onions, tomatoes, olives, and greens in tight rows on the third of the wrapper closest to you. Leave a half inch on each end empty. Tightly roll up the wrapper, tucking the ends in. Slice in half to serve.

MAKES 4 SERVINGS

BEANS

- 1 garlic clove, finely chopped
- ½ cup basil leaves, loosely packed
- ¼ cup extra-virgin olive oil
- 2 tablespoons balsamic vinegar
- 1½ cups precooked pinto beans, drained or 1 (15-ounce) can or carton
- ⅛ teaspoon cayenne pepper
- ¾ teaspoon sea salt
  Freshly ground black pepper

WRAP

- 4 (8-inch) whole-grain wraps or tortillas
- 2 avocados, pitted and thinly sliced
- ½ medium red onion, finely chopped
- 2 medium tomatoes, finely chopped and drained
- ½ cup Kalamata olives, pitted and halved
- 1 cup micro greens or finely chopped kale

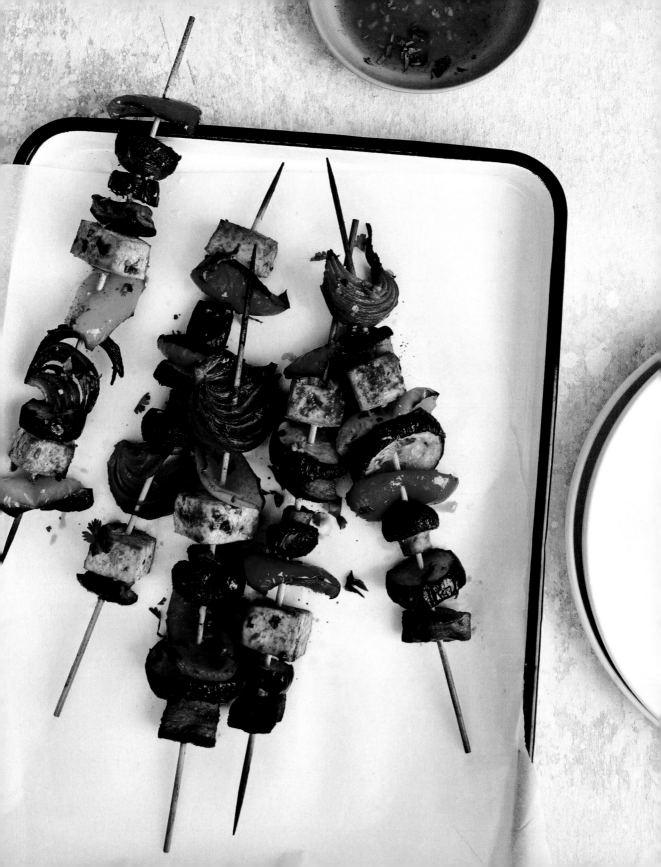

Colorful Kebab

These marinated kebabs are a great example of Health Is in the Hue. They're stacked with fresh, colorful vegetables, including purple eggplant, yellow and red bell peppers, red onions, mushrooms, and zucchini. They're perfect for oven-roasting at home or tossing on the grill at the next vegan cookout. The vegetables need to marinate for 1 hour prior to cooking, but you can use that time to prep Herbed Potato Salad (page 134) as a pairing.

MARINADE In a bowl, combine the marinade ingredients. Pour marinade in a deep baking pan with sides. Place the tofu and vegetables in a single layer in the marinade. Cover with plastic wrap and refrigerate for 1 hour, turning vegetables and tofu after 30 minutes.

ASSEMBLE AND COOK Preheat oven to 400°F.

Divide the tofu and vegetables among the eight skewers. Place skewers on a baking sheet lined with parchment paper and roast in the oven until the edges of the vegetables start to brown, about 10 minutes, checking often to make sure they don't burn. Turn the skewers so the uncooked side is closest to the heat and cook until the second side starts to brown, about 10 minutes. Serve hot.

MAKES 4 SERVINGS, 8 KEBABS

MARINADE

- ½ cup extra-virgin olive oil
- 6 garlic cloves, finely chopped
- ¼ cup freshly squeezed lime juice (about 2 limes)
- 1 teaspoon ground cumin
- 1 teaspoon smoked paprika
- ¼ cup chopped cilantro leaves
- 1½ teaspoons sea salt

KEBABS

- 1 block extra-firm tofu, cut into 16 or more cubes
- 8 white mushrooms (baby bella or white button)
- 1 small eggplant, sliced into ¼-inch cubes (about 8 or more)
- 1 red bell pepper, seeds removed, sliced into 8 pieces
- 1 yellow bell pepper, seeds removed, sliced into 8 pieces
- 1 orange bell pepper, seeds removed, sliced into 8 pieces
- 1 medium zucchini, sliced ¼ inch thick
- 1 medium red onion, sliced into 8 wedges
- 8 stainless steel or wooden skewers (if using wooden skewers, presoak them in water overnight)

PAD THAI

In this recipe, mounds of brown rice pad Thai noodles are tossed with crispy tofu and fresh vegetables, mixed with a spicy, lime-infused sauce, and topped with chopped peanuts. It's simple, flavorful, and delicious. It's also super nutritious—loaded with antioxidant-rich vegetables and protein-rich tofu and nuts.

SAUCE

- 2 tablespoons freshly squeezed lime juice (about 1 lime)
- ¼ cup coconut aminos or low-sodium tamari
- ¼ cup rice vinegar
- 1–2 tablespoons hot sauce

NOODLES

- 1 (8-ounce) package brown rice pad Thai noodles, cooked 2 minutes less than directed by package, to al dente
- 1 tablespoon sesame oil
- ½ teaspoon sea salt

TOFU

- 1 tablespoon sesame oil
- 1 pound extra-firm tofu, cut into ½-inch cubes
  Pinch sea salt

VEGETABLES

- 2 tablespoons extra-virgin coconut oil
- ¼ medium red onion, thinly sliced
- 3 garlic cloves, finely chopped
- 2 cups small broccoli florets
- ¼ teaspoon sea salt
- ¼ cup chopped cilantro leaves
- ½ medium-size head red cabbage, shredded (about 2 cups)
- 1 large carrot, grated
- 1 cup bean sprouts

GARNISH

- ⅓ cup chopped dry-roasted, unsalted peanuts
  Lime wedges

SAUCE In a small bowl, combine the sauce ingredients and set aside.

NOODLES In a medium bowl, toss the noodles with the oil and salt.

TOFU In a large skillet, heat the oil over medium-high heat. Stir in the tofu, sprinkle on salt, and sauté until golden brown on all sides, 5 to 10 minutes. Remove from the pan and set aside.

VEGETABLES In a large skillet, heat the oil over medium heat. Stir in the onions and garlic, and sauté until the onions are translucent, 3 to 5 minutes. Then add broccoli and salt. Sauté for 3 to 5 more minutes or until broccoli is tender. Add noodles and half of the sauce. Sauté for 3 more minutes, tossing constantly. Add the remainder of the sauce and simmer until noodles are hot, about 3 more minutes. Then add tofu, cilantro, cabbage, carrots, and bean sprouts and toss until incorporated, then remove from the heat.

GARNISH Top with peanuts and serve with lime wedges on the side.

MAKES 4 SERVINGS

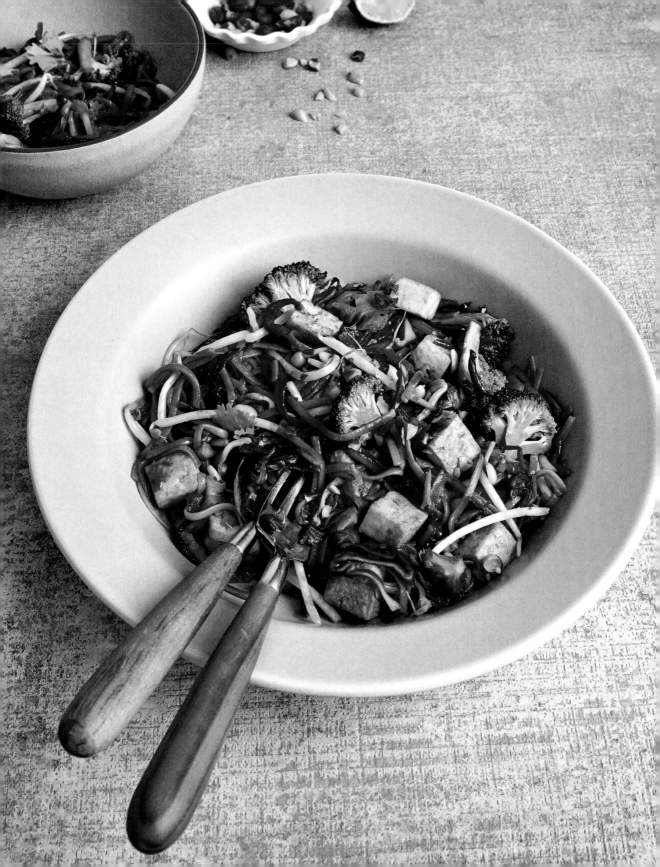

Buckwheat Soba Bowl

These buckwheat flour soba noodles have a chewy, nutty texture that complements the crunchy edamame and zesty miso sauce. The edamame also provides added protein, calcium, and iron to this fiber-rich and heart-healthy whole-grain dish. It's light, healthy, and satisfying, and equally delicious served warm or cold.

NOODLES

- 1 (8-ounce) package buckwheat soba noodles, cooked according to package directions
- 1 cup frozen edamame, cooked according to package directions
- 1 tablespoon sesame oil
- ½ teaspoon sea salt
- Freshly ground black pepper, to taste

VEGETABLES

- 1 medium carrot, shredded (about 1 cup)
- ¼ medium-size head purple cabbage, shredded (about 1½ cups)
- 2 tablespoons rice vinegar
- ¼ teaspoon sea salt

DRESSING

- 2 tablespoons sesame oil
- 2 tablespoons rice vinegar
- 1 tablespoon peeled and grated ginger
- 2 tablespoons miso (red, yellow, or white)

GARNISH

- Cilantro leaves
- Hot sauce, to taste

NOODLES In a large bowl, combine noodles with edamame, oil, salt, and pepper and set aside.

VEGETABLES In a second bowl, combine carrots and cabbage and season with rice vinegar and salt.

DRESSING In a blender, combine the dressing ingredients with ¼ cup water. Blend until very smooth.

ASSEMBLE AND GARNISH To assemble, toss the noodle mixture and the carrot mixture together in a large bowl. You can either drizzle the miso dressing on the noodles or serve it on the side. Garnish the noodles with cilantro and hot sauce.

MAKES 4 SERVINGS

AGELESS ANTIOXIDANTS   BRAIN BOOSTER   HEALTH IS IN THE HUE   LONGEVITY LOVER
PROTEIN DREAM   SMOOTH SKIN   STRONG BONES   SUPER GREENS   VISION MISSION

PEACH BBQ TEMPEH

Like tofu, tempeh takes on the flavor of the seasonings that are added to it. In this recipe, it's the sweet, citrusy, savory, and spicy taste of peach barbecue sauce that makes this protein-packed tempeh so good. This dish pairs well with Herbed Potato Salad (page 134) and Braised Sesame Kale (page 166).

Cut tempeh into ½-inch wide strips and place in a pan. Cover with ¾ cup water and simmer on low heat for 10 minutes. Drain with a slotted spoon, place on a dry plate, and season with salt and pepper.

Heat the oil in a large, heavy bottom skillet over medium-high heat. Add the tempeh and cook until brown, about 10 minutes on each side, using a spatula to gently flip the tempeh.

In a large bowl, gently mix the remaining ingredients together. Pour the sauce mixture over the tempeh in the skillet. Reduce the heat, cover, and simmer until most of the liquid evaporates, about 15 minutes. Serve immediately.

MAKES 4 SERVINGS

1 (8-ounce) package plain tempeh
½ teaspoon sea salt
Freshly ground black pepper, to taste
2 tablespoons extra-virgin olive oil
¼ onion, thinly sliced
2 peaches, peeled and finely chopped
1 garlic clove, finely chopped
1 teaspoon peeled and finely chopped ginger
2 tablespoons unsulphured molasses
1 tablespoon whole-grain mustard
2 tablespoons low-sodium tamari
1 tablespoon white vinegar
Cayenne, to taste

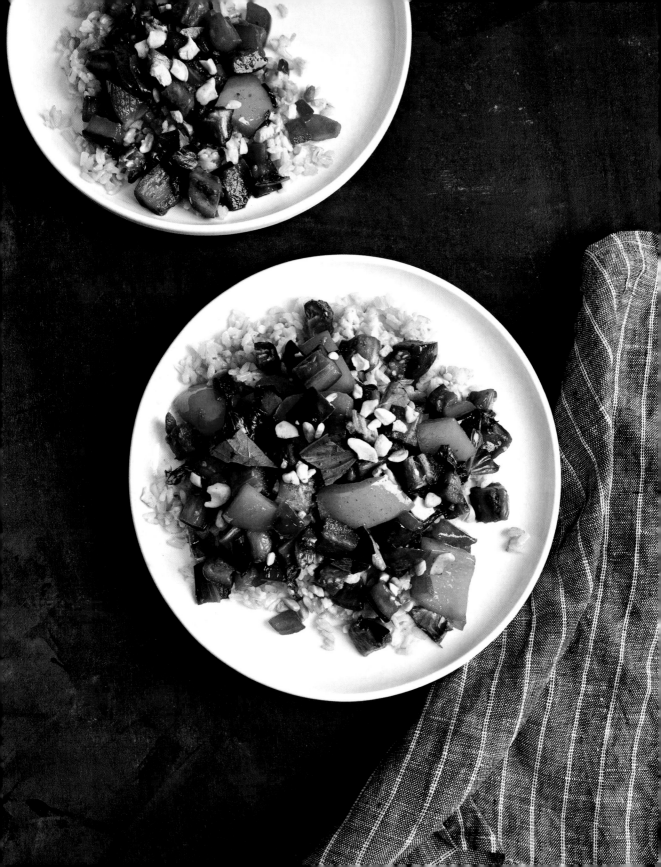

SPICY BASIL EGGPLANT
with DATES, CASHEWS, AND BROWN RICE

This colorful, antioxidant-rich eggplant dish has layers of texture and flavor in every mouthful. Spicy mixed vegetables combine with a tangy, savory sauce over fluffy brown rice. And they're topped with dates and cashews for an unexpected sweetness and crunchiness that are a perfect complement to the dish.

In a large pot, bring 2 cups water and rice to a boil. Reduce the heat, cover, and simmer for 45 minutes. Set cooked rice aside. In a large skillet, heat 2 teaspoons of the oil over medium-high heat. Add the eggplant cubes, sprinkle with a pinch of sea salt, and sauté until the cubes are tender, 2 to 3 minutes. Remove the eggplant cubes from the pan and set aside.

In the same skillet, heat the remaining 2 teaspoons of oil over medium-high heat. Stir in the onions, garlic, and ginger and sauté until the onions are translucent, 3 to 5 minutes. Add the bell pepper and sauté until the peppers are softened, 1 to 2 minutes. Add the eggplant cubes, vinegar, coconut aminos, and cayenne. Gently toss for 2 to 3 minutes. Taste and adjust seasonings, as desired. Remove pan from heat and toss in the basil. Serve hot over brown rice and topped with dates and cashews.

MAKES 4 SERVINGS

1 cup uncooked long-grain brown rice

4 teaspoons sesame oil

1 large purple eggplant, cut into bite-size cubes (about 4 to 5 cups)

Pinch sea salt

1 medium red onion, diced

6 garlic cloves, diced

½-inch piece ginger, peeled and chopped

1 orange or red bell pepper, seeds removed, chopped

1 tablespoon white or coconut vinegar or freshly squeezed lemon juice (about ½ lemon)

2 tablespoons coconut aminos or low-sodium tamari

¼ teaspoon cayenne

1 cup loosely packed basil leaves, chopped

10 Medjool dates, pitted and chopped

½ cup chopped cashews

STUFFED ORANGE AND RED
BELL PEPPERS

This dish was inspired by the delicious stuffed peppers we ate when I was growing up. This updated recipe uses a medley of wild rice, zucchini, walnuts, and currants for the filling and a cashew butter–based dressing on top. It's a great example of Health Is in the Hue because it contains antioxidant-rich foods in a variety of health-promoting colors.

FILLING

- ¾ cup uncooked wild rice
- 1 small zucchini, grated (about 2 cups)
- 1 cup raw walnuts, roughly chopped
- ¼ red onion, finely chopped (about ½ cup)
- ½ cup currants
- 3 tablespoons extra-virgin olive oil
- ¾ teaspoon sea salt
- Freshly ground black pepper, to taste
- 2 large red bell peppers, cut in half and seeds removed
- 2 large orange bell peppers, cut in half and seeds removed

SAUCE

- ¼ cup cashew butter
- ¼ cup freshly squeezed lemon juice (about 2 lemons)
- 2 tablespoons tahini
- 1 garlic clove, finely chopped
- 1 tablespoon nutritional yeast
- 1 tablespoon roughly chopped curly parsley
- 1 tablespoon roughly chopped fresh mint
- ½ teaspoon sea salt
- ⅛ teaspoon cayenne pepper
- Freshly ground black pepper, to taste
- 1 small cucumber, finely chopped (about 1 cup)

FILLING Preheat oven to 375°F.

Line a baking sheet with parchment paper and set aside.

Place the uncooked wild rice in a fine strainer and rinse. In a large pot, boil 4 cups water and the rice. Reduce the heat, cover, and simmer for 45 minutes and check for doneness. Some varieties of wild rice take longer to cook than others. The rice should be tender but still chewy, with some of the grains open. If not done, cover and continue simmering for another 10 to 15 minutes, if necessary. Once rice is done, drain off any remaining water.

In a large bowl, combine the cooked wild rice, zucchini, walnuts, onions, currants, oil, salt, and pepper.

Stuff the bell peppers with the wild rice mixture and place on the lined baking sheet. Bake for 45 minutes.

SAUCE In a blender, combine the cashew butter, lemon juice, ¼ cup water, tahini, garlic, nutritional yeast, parsley, mint, salt, cayenne, and pepper. Blend until smooth. Stir in the cucumbers. Serve stuffed bell peppers with the cucumber sauce on the side.

MAKES 4 SERVINGS

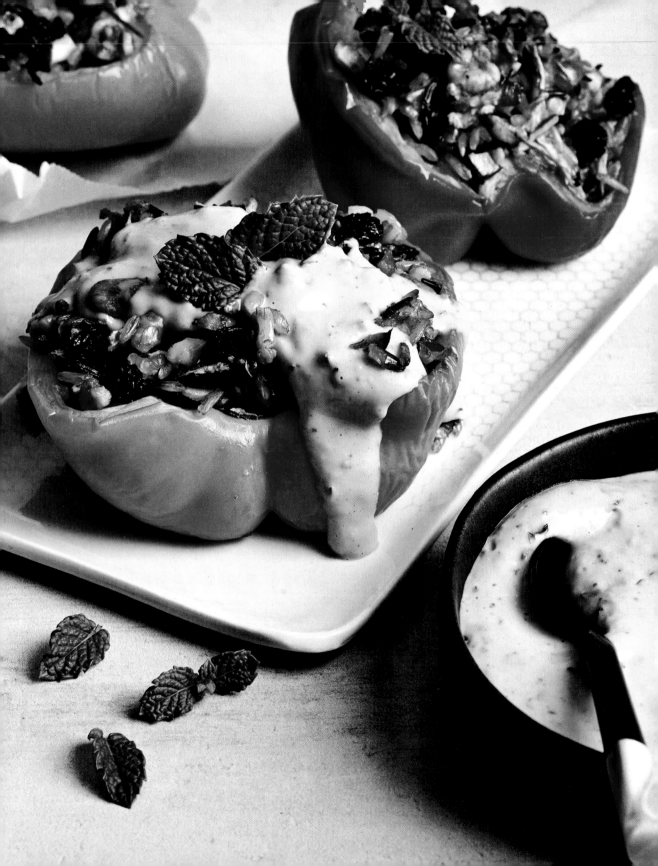

LASAGNA
with MUSHROOMS, EGGPLANT, AND ZUCCHINI

Rich, delicious, nutritious, and satisfying, this lasagna is a complete, balanced, all-in-one meal that impresses every time. And it's heart-healthy and cholesterol-free too!

1 pound extra-firm tofu, drained and pressed (see directions)

2 tablespoons plus 1 teaspoon extra-virgin olive oil

1 medium red onion, chopped

6 garlic cloves, chopped

1 pound white button mushrooms, chopped

1 cup Kalamata olives, pitted and chopped

3 tablespoons low-sodium tamari

2 tablespoons nutritional yeast

½ teaspoon dried oregano

½ teaspoon cayenne pepper

1 medium zucchini, halved and thinly sliced into half-moons

½ eggplant, thinly sliced and chopped

1 (12-ounce) package whole-grain lasagna noodles

2 (24-ounce) jars of tomato sauce

1 bunch fresh spinach, chopped (about 4 cups, packed)

1 cup basil leaves, torn

Preheat oven to 350°F.

Squeeze the excess water out of the tofu by pressing it in a towel. In a large bowl, crumble the tofu with a fork.

Heat 2 teaspoons of the oil in a large skillet over medium heat. Add the onions, garlic, and mushrooms and sauté until the mushrooms are soft, about 3 to 5 minutes. Drain any liquid and add the mushroom mixture to the crumbled tofu. Add the olives, tamari, nutritional yeast, oregano, and cayenne. Stir until well mixed. Adjust seasonings to make this spicy. Set aside to marinate.

In the same skillet, heat 1 teaspoon of oil over medium heat. Add the zucchini and sauté until soft, 5 to 7 minutes. Place in a bowl and set aside.

In the same skillet, heat 1 teaspoon of oil over medium heat. Add the eggplant and sauté until soft, 3 to 5 minutes. Combine the eggplant with the zucchini and set aside.

Cook the lasagna noodles half the time stated on the package.

Spread the remaining 1 tablespoon of oil over the bottom of a large casserole dish and then cover the oil with a layer of tomato sauce. Place a layer of noodles on top of the sauce. Spread half the tofu mixture over the noodles. Next, add a layer of spinach to cover the tofu and then add half the basil leaves on top of the spinach. Layer the zucchini mixture on top of the basil. Add another layer of noodles and cover them with another layer of sauce. Add the remaining tofu mixture, then spinach, then basil leaves, then zucchini mixture. Cover with a final layer of noodles and sauce. Cover with foil and bake for 45 minutes. Serve hot.

MAKES 8-10 SERVINGS

ENCHILADAS

These protein-rich enchiladas are stuffed with squash, black beans, and corn, and layered with a spicy, smoky, chipotle pepper and tomato sauce. Topped with avocado slices, salsa, and sour cream, this dish is hearty and satisfying.

SQUASH Preheat oven to 375°F.

Line a baking sheet with parchment paper. Cut squash in half and discard the seeds. Rub squash, both the flesh and the skin, with oil. Place on the lined baking sheet cut side down and bake until soft, about 30 minutes. Remove flesh with a spoon, place in a bowl, and mash with the back of a fork.

SAUCE In a blender, combine the sauce ingredients and blend together.

ENCHILADAS Preheat oven to 425°F.

In a large bowl, mix the squash, black beans, corn, oil, and salt until thoroughly combined.

ASSEMBLE In a 13 x 9-inch ovenproof baking dish, spread ¾ cup of the tomato sauce. Next, stuff each tortilla with about ½ cup of the squash mixture, roll, and place closely next to each other in the baking dish on the tomato sauce with the ends facing down. Pour remaining sauce over the enchiladas and bake for 40 minutes.

SALSA In a medium bowl, combine the salsa ingredients. Serve hot enchiladas topped with the salsa, avocado, and sour cream.

MAKES 4 SERVINGS

SQUASH

- 2 small acorn squashes or 1 large butternut squash
- 1 tablespoon extra-virgin olive oil

SAUCE

- 1 (25-ounce) jar peeled whole or crushed tomatoes
- 1 tablespoon extra-virgin olive oil
- 2 garlic cloves, finely chopped
- 1 tablespoon ground chipotle peppers
- ½ teaspoon sea salt

ENCHILADAS

- 1½ cups precooked black beans or 1 (15-ounce) can or carton
- 1 cup corn, fresh or cooked from frozen according to package instructions
- 1 tablespoon extra-virgin olive oil
- ½ teaspoon sea salt
- 8 (8-inch) whole grain tortillas

SALSA

- 2 medium tomatoes, diced
- ¼ cup finely chopped cilantro
- ¼ medium red onion, finely diced
- 2 teaspoons freshly squeezed lime juice (about ⅓ lime)
- 1–2 jalapeños, to taste
- ½ teaspoon sea salt

TOPPING

- 1 avocado, pitted and thinly sliced
  Cashew Sour Cream (page 102)

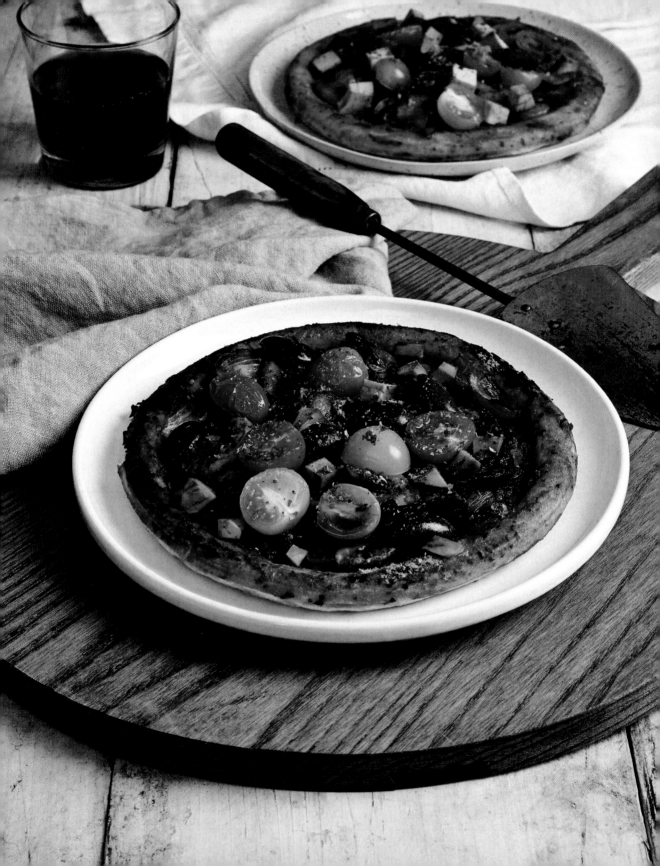

BASIL MUSHROOM PIZZA

Friday night pizza just got better—no dairy or vegan cheese required! Fresh and flavorful ingredients like mushrooms, olives, basil, and avocado sprinkled with nutritional yeast and cayenne pepper take this pizza to a healthier, tastier level.

Preheat oven to 350°F.

If pizza crust dough is frozen, let it thaw. Brush the thawed crust with tomato sauce. Sprinkle on nutritional yeast to cover sauce. Bake pizza crust for 10 to 12 minutes or until edges of crust begin to turn golden brown.

Heat the oil in a large skillet over medium heat. Add the onions, garlic, mushrooms, and coconut aminos and sauté until the mushrooms are soft, 3 to 5 minutes. Remove the pizza crust from the oven. Using a slotted spoon to drain the liquid, arrange the mushroom mixture on top of the pizza crust. Arrange tomatoes, olives, avocado, and basil on top of mushroom mixture. Sprinkle cayenne pepper on top. Bake 5 more minutes or until toppings are heated enough for your taste. Serve hot.

MAKES 3-4 SERVINGS

1 prepared whole-grain pizza crust

3–4 tablespoons tomato sauce

2 tablespoons nutritional yeast

2 teaspoons extra-virgin olive oil

¼ large red onion, chopped

3 garlic cloves, peeled and chopped

1 cup white button mushrooms, thinly sliced

2 teaspoons coconut aminos or low-sodium tamari

1 pint cherry tomatoes, halved

2 tablespoons Kalamata olives, pitted and halved

2 avocados, pitted and chopped into cubes

½ cup loosely packed fresh basil, finely chopped

½ teaspoon cayenne pepper, or to taste

VEGETABLE STIR-FRY
with BLACK RICE AND ALMOND BUTTER SAUCE

Thick and creamy almond butter takes this dish from simple to sublime. And the colorful variety of foods reflect a range of powerful health-promoting antioxidants. The broccoli and brown rice contain vision-protecting compounds that help prevent cataracts and macular degeneration. And the almonds and almond butter add vital protein to round out the meal.

BLACK RICE

- 1 cup uncooked black rice
- 2 teaspoons sesame oil
- ¼ teaspoon salt

VEGETABLES

- 1 tablespoon extra-virgin coconut oil
- 1 tablespoon peeled and finely chopped ginger
- 2 garlic cloves, finely chopped
- 2 cups broccoli florets (from about 1 large head of broccoli)
- ½ medium head bok choy, both leaves and white part, thinly sliced into strips (about 2 cups)
- 1 pound asparagus, remove and discard ends
- 2 cups snow peas, tips removed
- 1 red bell pepper, seeds removed, thinly sliced
- ½ teaspoon salt

SAUCE

- ⅓ cup raw almond butter
- 2 tablespoons rice vinegar
- 2 tablespoons coconut aminos or low-sodium tamari
- ⅛ teaspoon cayenne pepper, or more to taste

GARNISH

- ¼ cup chopped raw almonds
- Hot sauce

BLACK RICE In a large pot, add the rice and 2 cups water and bring to a boil. Reduce the heat, cover, and simmer for 45 minutes. Remove the pan from the heat and let it sit for 10 minutes covered to finish cooking. Fluff the rice with a fork and season with oil and salt.

VEGETABLES In a large skillet, heat the oil over medium heat. Stir in the ginger and garlic and sauté until fragrant, about 1 minute. Add broccoli, bok choy, and asparagus. Sauté for 3 to 5 minutes or until the broccoli istender. Add the snow peas, bell pepper, and salt, and sauté for 3 more minutes.

SAUCE In a small bowl, combine the sauce ingredients with 2 tablespoons water and stir until smooth. Add the sauce to the vegetable mixture and toss until thoroughly incorporated.

SERVE Place the vegetables over the rice and top with the almonds. Serve with hot sauce on the side. This stir-fry also tastes great with Crispy Tofu Bites (page 111) tossed in.

MAKES 4 SERVINGS

AGELESS ANTIOXIDANTS BRAIN BOOSTER HEALTH IS IN THE HUE LONGEVITY LOVER
PROTEIN DREAM SMOOTH SKIN STRONG BONES SUPER GREENS VISION MISSION

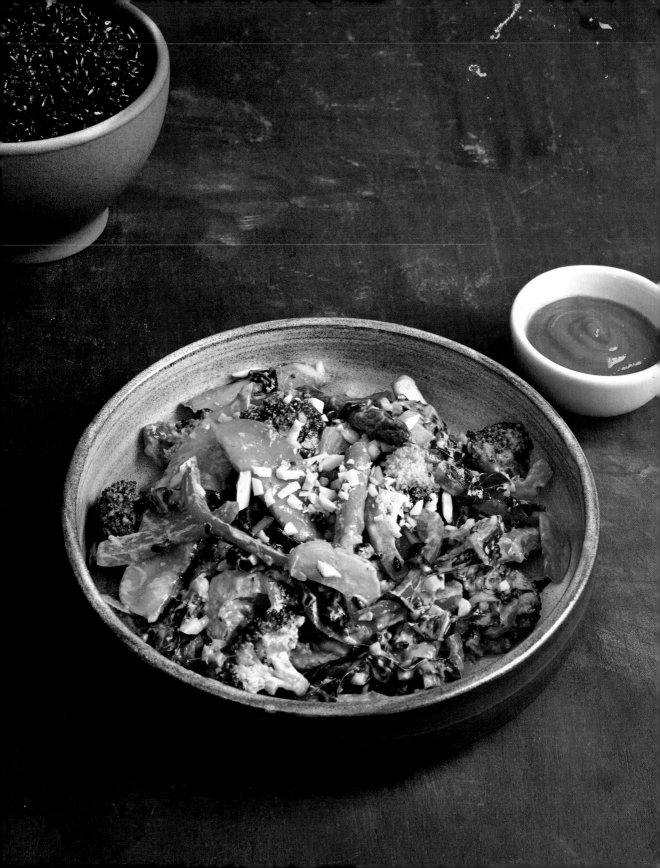

Roasted Sweet Potato
and Black Bean Bowl
with LIME CILANTRO VINAIGRETTE

I love one-bowl meals and this recipe fits the bill perfectly. In addition to sweet potatoes and black beans, this bowl brims with corn and quinoa and a chipotle-spiced lime cilantro vinaigrette drizzled on top. These ingredients also taste great in a warm tortilla or over a bed of dark leafy greens.

QUINOA

- 1 cup red quinoa
- 2 cups pea shoots or arugula
- 1 tablespoon extra-virgin olive oil
- 1 teaspoon freshly squeezed lime juice (about ¼ lime)
- ½ teaspoon sea salt

SWEET POTATOES

- 1 large unpeeled sweet potato, diced (about 2 cups)
- 2 teaspoons extra-virgin olive oil
- ¼ teaspoon sea salt

BLACK BEANS AND CORN

- 1½ cups precooked black beans or 1 (15-ounce) can or carton
- 1 cup corn, fresh or cooked from frozen according to package instructions
- 1 tablespoon finely chopped red onion
- 2 teaspoons extra-virgin olive oil
- ¼ teaspoon cumin
- ¼ teaspoon sea salt

LIME CILANTRO VINAIGRETTE

- ¼ cup extra-virgin olive oil
- ¼ cup cilantro leaves
- 2 tablespoons freshly squeezed lime juice (about 1 lime)
- ¼ teaspoon sea salt
- ¼ teaspoon chipotle powder
- 1 avocado, pitted and thinly sliced, for garnish

RECIPE CONTINUED ON PAGE 196

AGELESS ANTIOXIDANTS   BRAIN BOOSTER   HEALTH IS IN THE HUE   LONGEVITY LOVER
PROTEIN DREAM   SMOOTH SKIN   STRONG BONES   SUPER GREENS   VISION MISSION

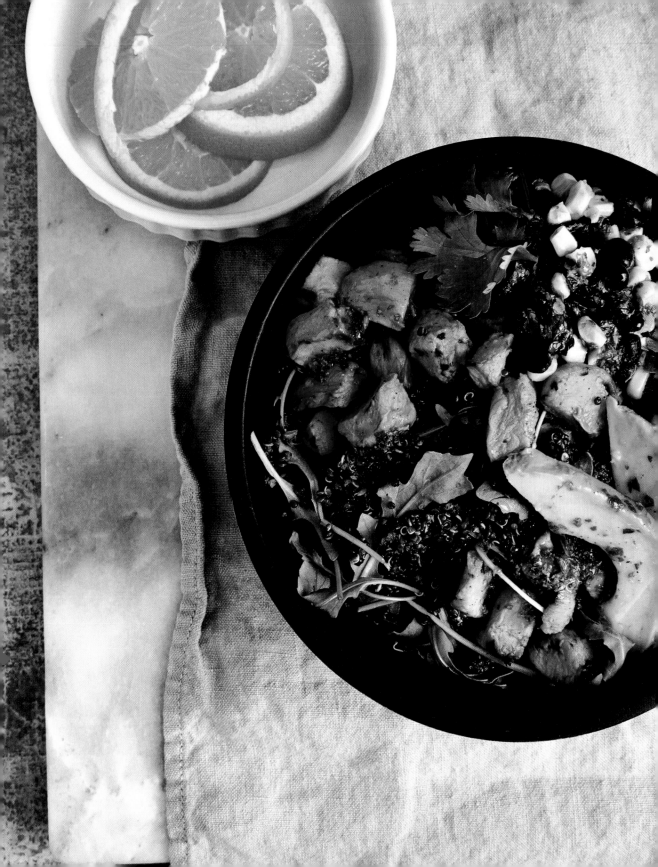

RECIPE CONTINUED FROM PAGE 194

Preheat oven to 375°F.

QUINOA In a large pot, bring 2 cups water and quinoa to a boil. Reduce the heat, cover, and simmer until all the water evaporates, about 15 minutes. Remove from heat and keep covered for 5 minutes. In a medium bowl, combine the quinoa, greens, oil, lime juice, and salt.

SWEET POTATOES Line a baking sheet with parchment paper. Place sweet potatoes in a bowl and coat with oil and salt. Place on the lined baking sheet and bake until tender and browned, about 20 minutes.

BLACK BEANS AND CORN In a medium bowl, combine the beans, corn, onion, oil, cumin, and salt. Toss until thoroughly combined.

VINAIGRETTE Combine the oil, cilantro, lime juice, salt, and chipotle powder in a blender and process until smooth.

ASSEMBLE In four individual serving bowls, arrange the sweet potatoes, beans mixture, quinoa mixture, and avocado. Drizzle with the vinaigrette and serve the extra sauce on the side.

MAKES 4 SERVINGS

CURRIED CHICKPEAS
in WARM PITA POCKET

These protein-powered curried chickpeas are seriously delicious. The creamy sauce, spicy seasonings, fresh vegetables, and chewy chickpeas are the perfect combination. They make a light yet satisfying lunch as the filling for a warm, whole-grain pita.

Preheat oven to 350°F.

In a large bowl, mix the chickpeas with all the other ingredients, except pita, arugula, and avocado. Let the ingredients marinate for 15 minutes. Place the pita halves on a baking sheet lined with parchment paper and warm for about 5 minutes. The bread should be warm, not toasted. Place ¼ cup of arugula in the bottom of each pita half. Next, using a slotted spoon to drain excess liquid, place the chickpeas inside the pita pockets. Top with avocados and serve immediately.

MAKES 4 SERVINGS

2   (15-ounce) cans or cartons chickpeas
1   small red onion, chopped
4   garlic cloves, chopped
1   teaspoon curry powder
1   tablespoon nutritional yeast
1   red bell pepper, seeds removed, chopped
2   tablespoons Kalamata olives, pitted and halved
5   leaves fresh basil, chopped
1   tablespoon grapeseed oil or vegan mayo
2   tablespoons coconut aminos or low-sodium tamari
4   whole-grain pitas, halved (you will have 8 pita halves)
2   cups arugula
1   avocado, pitted and chopped

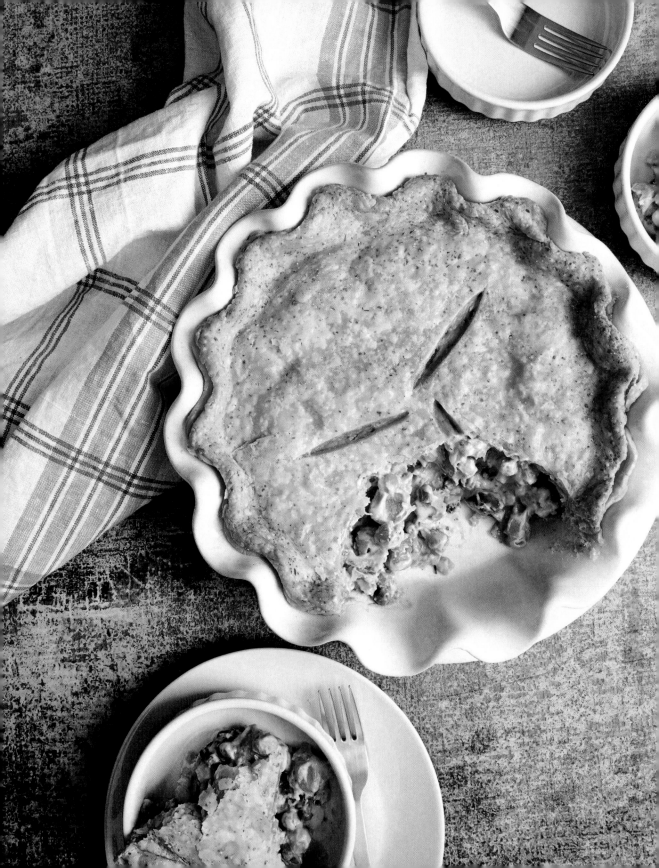

VEGETABLE POT PIE

Vegetable pot pie was one of the only ways my mother could get me to eat my vegetables with glee when I was growing up. The vegetables were smothered in a thick, creamy sauce between two pie crusts. What's not to love? Well, this recipe is a healthier version of those pot pies I loved as a child. The sauce is now made with coconut milk and nutritional yeast, and the filling of colorful, antioxidant-rich mixed vegetables has protein-packed chickpeas added in. Still an awesome way to eat my veggies!

Preheat oven to 375°F.

In a large soup pot, heat the oil over medium heat. Stir in the onions and garlic, and sauté until the onions are translucent, about 3 minutes. Add mushrooms and sauté for another 3 minutes. Add the milk, flour, nutritional yeast, salt, thyme, and cayenne, and mix until thoroughly combined. Reduce the heat, cover, and simmer for 5 minutes, stirring often. Place the vegetable mixture in a large bowl and stir in frozen vegetables and chickpeas. Stir in black pepper, taste, and adjust seasonings, as desired. Spoon the filling into the bottom pie crust. Cover the filling with the top pie crust, cut away the excess crust, and crimp the edges of the crusts together to seal. Make three small slits in the top center. Lightly brush the pie crust with coconut oil. Bake 35 to 40 minutes or until crust turns golden brown. Let cool for about 10 minutes before serving. The pot pie can be stored in the freezer in an airtight container for up to 3 months.

MAKES 6-8 SERVINGS

2   tablespoons extra-virgin olive oil

1   yellow onion, diced

3   garlic cloves, finely chopped

½   cup finely chopped mushrooms

1   (13.5-ounce) can coconut milk (light or regular)

1   tablespoon whole wheat flour

3   tablespoons nutritional yeast

2   teaspoons sea salt

1   teaspoon thyme

¼   teaspoon cayenne pepper

2   cups frozen mixed vegetables (carrots, corn, peas, and green beans)

1   (13.5-ounce) can or carton chickpeas, drained

Freshly ground black pepper, to taste

2   (9-inch) frozen prepared whole-grain pie crusts, thawed

1   tablespoon extra-virgin coconut oil, melted

SAVORY VEGETABLE QUICHE

This cholesterol-free quiche is simply scrumptious—it's perfectly textured, well seasoned, and loaded with fresh green vegetables. Enjoy it for any meal of the day—lunch, dinner, breakfast, or brunch. Or bring it to your next potluck. It makes a pretty dish for any occasion.

CRUST
- 1 (9-inch) whole-grain pie crust

FILLING
- 1 block firm tofu, drained and pressed (see directions)
- 3 tablespoons nutritional yeast
- 2 teaspoons oregano
- ½ teaspoon sea salt

VEGETABLES
- 2 tablespoons extra-virgin olive oil
- 2 small leeks or 1 large leek, thinly sliced, white part only (about 1 cup)
- 3 garlic cloves, finely chopped
- 4 medium zucchinis or 2 large zucchinis, thinly sliced, about ⅛ inch thick
- 1 teaspoon sea salt
- Cayenne pepper, to taste
- Freshly ground black pepper, to taste
- 2 cups baby spinach
- ½ cup basil leaves, loosely packed

CRUST Preheat oven to 375°F.

Thaw pie crust for 10 minutes. Place the crust in the oven for 10 minutes and then set aside.

FILLING Squeeze the excess water out of the tofu by pressing it in a towel. Place the tofu, nutritional yeast, oregano, and salt in a food processor and process until smooth.

VEGETABLES In a large skillet, heat the oil over medium heat. Stir in the leeks and garlic, and sauté until the leeks are translucent, 3 to 5 minutes, stirring often. Add zucchini, salt, cayenne, and pepper, stirring often until the zucchini is tender, about 5 minutes, then remove from heat. Place zucchini mixture in a large bowl and stir in the spinach, basil, and tofu mixture. Taste and adjust seasoning, as desired. Spoon the filling into the pie crust; smooth out with the back of a spoon. Bake until firm, about 35 minutes, then let sit for at least 10 minutes before slicing. Serve warm or at room temperature.

MAKES 6-8 SERVINGS

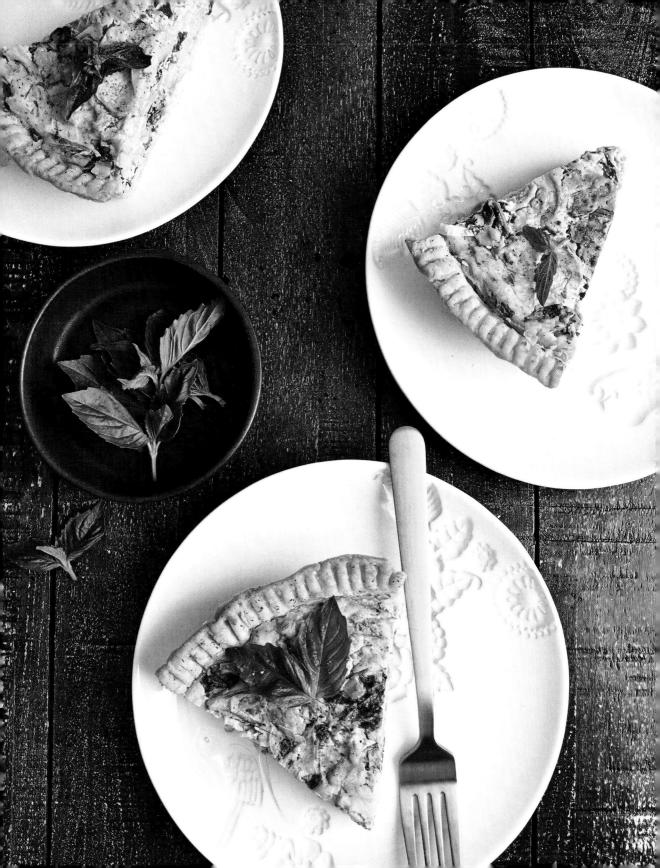

ETHIOPIAN PLATTER

When we first went vegan all those years ago, we went to Ethiopian restaurants often because they had so many vegan options and the food was fabulous. To this day, Ethiopian food is still one of our favorite cuisines. So of course, we had to include a traditionally inspired Ethiopian platter among the recipes. There's lots of vegetable chopping in this recipe, but I promise you, it's worth it. In fact, invite some friends over and make it together. It'll taste even better that way!

COLLARD GREENS

- 1 tablespoon extra-virgin olive oil
- ¼ medium yellow onion, sliced
- 3 garlic cloves, finely chopped
- 1 bunch collard greens, stems removed and greens chopped in thin ribbons (about 4 cups)
- ½ teaspoon sea salt

CABBAGE, POTATO, AND CARROT

- 1 tablespoon extra-virgin olive oil
- ½ medium yellow onion, chopped
- 2 garlic cloves, finely chopped
- 1 jalapeño, chopped
- ¼ teaspoon cumin
- ½ teaspoon turmeric
- ¼ teaspoon ground cardamom
- ¼ teaspoon cinnamon
- ¼ teaspoon ground clove
- 1 medium carrot, chopped into ¼-inch slices (about 1 cup)
- 1 medium golden potato, chopped into ¼-inch slices (about 1 cup)
- ⅓ head cabbage, finely sliced (about 3 cups)
- ½ teaspoon sea salt

RED LENTILS

- 1 tablespoon extra-virgin olive oil
- ¼ medium yellow onion, finely chopped
- 2 teaspoons berbere spice (or more, to taste)
- 3 garlic cloves, finely chopped
- 1 cup uncooked red lentils
- ½ teaspoon sea salt

TOMATO SALAD

- 3 medium tomatoes, chopped (about 3 cups)
- 2 tablespoons finely chopped red onion
- 1–2 jalapeños, thinly sliced
- 3 tablespoons extra-virgin olive oil
- 2 tablespoons white wine vinegar
- 1 teaspoon peeled and grated ginger
- ½ teaspoon sea salt
- Freshly ground black pepper, to taste
- 4 whole-grain injeras

COLLARD GREENS In a large skillet, heat the oil over medium heat. Stir in the onions and garlic and sauté until the onions are translucent, 3 to 5 minutes. Add collard greens, ½ cup water, and salt. Cover and simmer until tender, about 10 minutes, stirring occasionally.

CABBAGE, POTATO, AND CARROT In a large skillet, heat the oil over medium heat. Stir in the onions, garlic, and jalapeño, and sauté until the onions are translucent, 3 to 5 minutes. Add the spices and stir until incorporated. Add the carrot, potato, cabbage, ¼ cup water, and salt and mix very well. Cover and cook, stirring every 5 minutes until potatoes are tender, about 15 minutes.

RED LENTILS In a large skillet, heat the oil over medium heat. Stir in the onions, and sauté until they are translucent, 3 to 5 minutes. Add the berbere and garlic and combine thoroughly. Add 3 cups water and stir until all the ingredients are combined. Add the lentils and salt and bring to a boil. Reduce heat and simmer until the lentils start to break apart, about 20 minutes.

TOMATO SALAD In a large bowl, combine the tomato, onion, and jalapeño. In a separate medium bowl, whisk together the oil, vinegar, ginger, salt, and pepper. Pour the sauce into the tomato mixture and combine thoroughly.

To serve, spread one piece of injera on a large plate. Spoon collard greens, cabbage, lentils, and tomato separately onto injera. Add extra injera on the side.

TIPS Injera, Ethiopia's traditional fermented flatbread made of nutritious teff flour, is available in some national grocery stores, in local Ethiopian grocery stores, and online. If you don't have injera, substitute whole-grain tortillas or pita.

Berbere, a traditional Ethiopian chili spice blend, is available at many grocery stores and online.

MAKES 4-6 SERVINGS

THREE-BEAN CHILI

This chili is a delicious way to eat a variety of beans at once, which is good news because eating beans every day is one of the keys to achieving optimal health and longevity. They're high in protein, fiber, iron, and other vital nutrients and can help prevent the risk of heart disease—our number-one cause of death. This recipe calls for pinto, kidney, and black beans, but any of your favorites will do. The chili tastes even better the next day, once the seasonings have had a chance to meld.

2 tablespoons olive oil

2 red onions, chopped

4 garlic cloves, chopped

1 tablespoon chili powder

1 teaspoon cumin

1 medium red bell pepper, seeds removed, diced ¼ inch thick

2 medium carrots, diced ¼ inch thick

1 stalk celery, diced ¼ inch thick

1 teaspoon basil

1 teaspoon oregano

1 teaspoon cayenne pepper

2 tablespoons chili flakes

1 (15-ounce) can no-sodium diced tomatoes

4 cups low-sodium vegetable broth or water

1½ cups precooked pinto beans or 1 (15-ounce) can or carton

1½ cups precooked kidney beans or 1 (15-ounce) can or carton

1½ cups precooked black beans or 1 (15-ounce) can or carton

1 teaspoon sea salt

Black pepper, to taste

1 tablespoon low-sodium tamari

1 teaspoon barley miso

In a large skillet, heat the oil over medium heat. Stir in the onions, garlic, chili powder, and cumin and sauté 3 to 5 minutes, stirring constantly. Add bell peppers, carrots, celery, basil, oregano, cayenne pepper, and chili pepper flakes and sauté for 3 more minutes, stirring occasionally. Stir in tomatoes and cook for 3 more minutes.

In a large pot, add the vegetable stock and the beans and bring to a boil. Turn heat to low. Stir the vegetable mixture into the pot of beans. Add salt, pepper, tamari, and miso. Taste and adjust seasonings, as desired. Simmer for 15 minutes. While the chili is simmering, scoop out 2 cups of the chili, place them in a food processor, and blend until smooth, about 1 minute. Place the blended chili back in the pot, stir, and continue simmering. Serve hot with Southern-Style Cornbread (page 128). This chili freezes well for batch cooking.

MAKES 10-12 SERVINGS

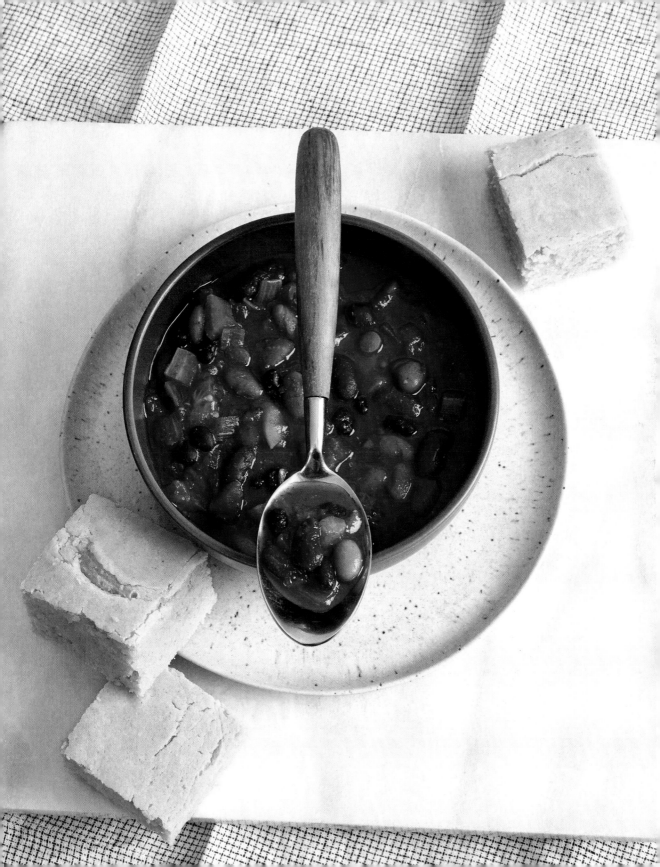

Desserts

For the desserts in this chapter, we use 100 percent whole grains and natural sweeteners. So they're healthier sweets you can feel good about eating. What a treat! If we had to pick our favorite dessert from this collection—and it wouldn't be easy—we'd have to go with Perfect Pecan Pie. It's absolutely divine, as you'll see! But all the desserts are scrumptious, from the No-Bake Chocolate Pie with Pistachios, Raspberry Cheesecake Tartlets, and Apple Crumb Pie to the baker's delight Fudge Walnut Brownies and Cakey Banana Chocolate Chip Cookies. We know you'll enjoy them as much as we do.

Cakey Banana Chocolate Chip Cookies

Macadamia Coconut Cacao Nib Brittle

Fudge Walnut Brownies

Hazelnut Date Bars

Peach Cobbler

Perfect Pecan Pie

Apple Crumb Pie

Maple Pecan Ice Cream

No-Bake Chocolate Pie with Pistachios

Raspberry Cheesecake Tartlets

Fruity Ice Pops

Pineapple Carrot Cupcakes with Orange Cashew Cream Topping

Almost Ambrosia

CAKEY BANANA
CHOCOLATE CHIP COOKIES

These cookies bake up soft and thick, with a cake-like interior. They're full of chocolate flavor, with hint of banana and the buttery crunch of pecans. And they're made with white whole wheat flour, which is 100 precent whole grain flour made from hard white wheat berries instead of the hard red wheat berries used for whole wheat flour.

1 very ripe banana

½ cup coconut sugar (depending on desired sweetness)

½ cup extra-virgin solid coconut oil

1 teaspoon vanilla extract

¼ cup unsweetened almond milk

2 cups white whole wheat flour

1 teaspoon baking soda

1 teaspoon baking powder

¼ teaspoon sea salt

1 cup semi-sweet mini chocolate chips

½ cup chopped pecans

Preheat oven to 350°F.

In a large bowl, mash the banana. Add the sugar, oil, vanilla, and milk until well combined. In a separate bowl, whisk together the flour, baking soda, baking powder, and salt. Add the dry mixture to the wet mixture until just combined. Fold in the chocolate chips and pecans.

Place rounded tablespoons of the cookie dough onto a baking sheet lined with parchment paper. Gently press down on the cookies until they are about ¼ inch thick and 2 inches in diameter. Bake for 10 to 12 minutes. Let cookies stay on the baking sheet for about 3 minutes to finish cooking and set. Then gently place them on a wire rack to cool completely. Serve with Vanilla Almond Milk (page 80).

TIP For sweeter cookies, use ¾ cup coconut sugar or 2 very ripe bananas.

MAKES 14-16 COOKIES

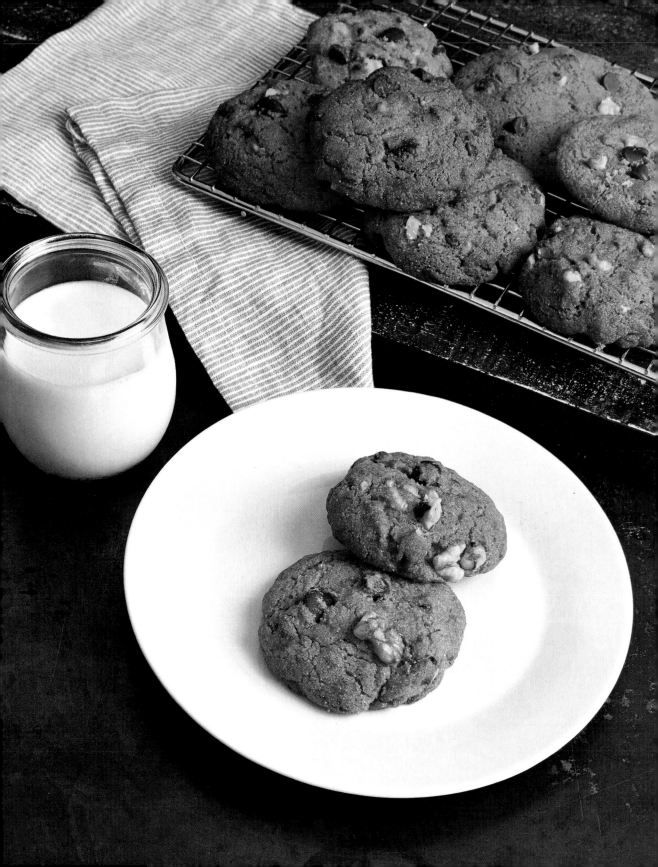

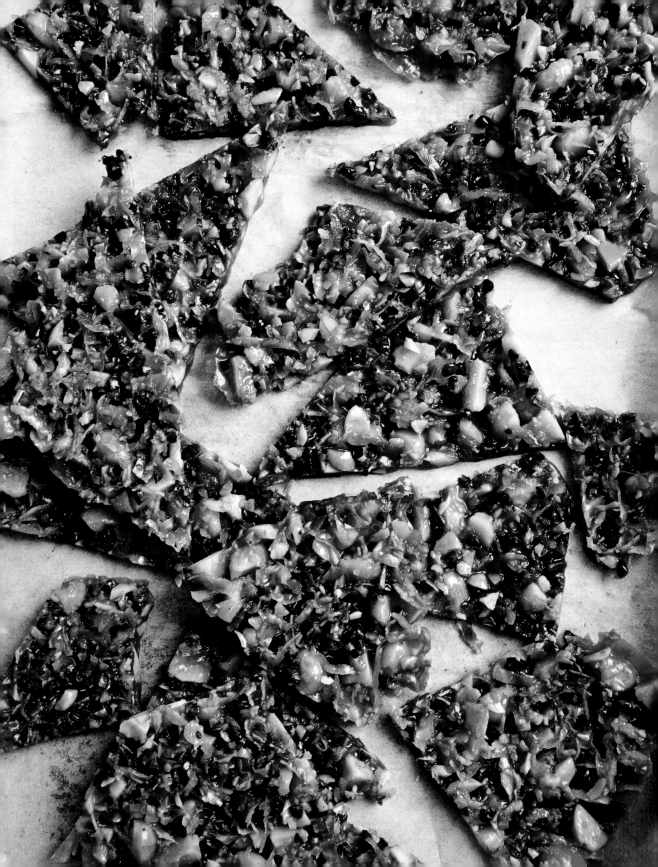

MACADAMIA
COCONUT CACAO NIB BRITTLE

Macadamia coconut cacao nib brittle—it's a mouthful to say, but delicious to eat. It's crunchy, nutty, buttery, and chocolatey—and made with only seven simple ingredients. Cacao nibs are the star ingredient. They're less refined versions of the cocoa used in most chocolate, so more of their nutrients are retained, including ageless antioxidants shown to improve cognitive function, reduce the risk of heart disease, and increase longevity. They're available in healthier food stores.

Preheat oven to 325°F.

Line a baking sheet with parchment paper. In a medium bowl, combine the nuts, coconut flakes, cacao nibs, sugar, and salt.

In a small pan, combine the oil and maple syrup. Simmer over medium heat until the ingredients are combined, about 3 minutes, stirring continuously until the edges bubble.

Pour the oil mixture over the nut mixture. Stir thoroughly and then pour the mixture onto the baking sheet. Smooth it out with the back of a spoon to spread it as evenly as possible.

Bake for 15 minutes, checking to be sure it doesn't overcook.

Place the baking sheet in the refrigerator until cool. Remove from the refrigerator and break the brittle into pieces. Serve immediately. To store, place wax paper in between layers of brittle in an airtight container and keep in a cool, dry place for up to 2 weeks.

MAKES 6 SERVINGS

1 cup coarsely chopped macadamia nuts

½ cup dried, unsweetened coconut flakes

¼ cup cacao nibs

2 tablespoons coconut sugar

Pinch sea salt

2 tablespoons extra-virgin coconut oil

½ cup maple syrup

FUDGE WALNUT BROWNIES

Moist, chewy, and chocolatey, these brownies are a healthier, indulgent treat.

¼ cup ground flaxseed meal

¼ cup raw almond butter

¾ cup coconut sugar

¼ cup maple syrup

¼ cup plus 2 tablespoons extra-virgin coconut oil, melted

¾ cup unsweetened cocoa powder

¼ teaspoon sea salt

¼ cup plus 2 tablespoons white whole wheat flour

¾ cup chopped walnuts

Preheat oven to 325°F.

In a small bowl, whisk together flaxseed meal and ¾ cup water and set aside. Line an 8 x 8-inch baking pan with parchment paper and set aside.

In a mixer, add almond butter, coconut sugar, maple syrup, and oil and mix well. Add cocoa powder slowly and continue to mix until batter is very smooth. Add the salt and flaxseed mixture and mix well. Slowly fold in the flour and mix well. Fold in the walnuts. Pour the batter into the baking pan and smooth using a rubber spatula. Bake until a toothpick inserted in the middle comes out nearly clean, 25 to 30 minutes. Unlike a cake, it should not be completely clean, but it should not be wet with batter. Cool completely, about 45 minutes. Cut into squares and serve.

TIP Add ¼ cup more coconut sugar for sweeter brownies.

MAKES 16 BROWNIES

HAZELNUT DATE BARS

We love nuts and dried fruits and these raw bars that my mom created are a healthy treat that's full of protein. The rich flavors of hazelnuts and apricots really stand out. They're perfect to keep in your food stash (as we talk about on page 43). Just wrap the bars individually and store them in the refrigerator to grab and go.

Line the bottom of an 8 x 8-inch baking pan with parchment paper. Place the whole almonds in a food processor and process until a soft almond butter is formed. Place the banana in a blender and blend for 1 minute. Add the raisins and apricots and blend for 1 more minute.

In a large bowl, combine the almond butter, fruit mixture, and the chopped almonds, hazelnuts, pecans, walnuts, dates, figs, and ¼ cup of the coconut. Mix ingredients well with a spoon. Press the mixture into the pan. Sprinkle the remaining coconut on top. Chill in the refrigerator for 30 minutes to firm. Cut into squares and serve.

MAKES 10-12 SERVINGS

- ½ cup raw whole almonds
- 1 ripe banana
- ½ cup raisins
- ½ cup dried apricots
- 1 cup raw almonds, coarsely chopped
- 1 cup hazelnuts, coarsely chopped
- 1 cup pecans, coarsely chopped
- 1 cup walnuts, coarsely chopped
- 5 Medjool dates, pitted and chopped
- 4 Calimyrna figs, chopped
- ½ cup unsweetened shredded coconut

PEACH COBBLER

This easy-to-make cobbler has ripe, juicy peaches on the bottom and a sweet biscuit crust on top. A wholesome and delicious dessert, the peaches are high in antioxidant vitamin C, which can help improve overall skin texture and reduce wrinkling.

CRUST

- 1½ cups white whole wheat flour, sifted
- ¼ cup coconut sugar
- 1 teaspoon baking powder
- ½ teaspoon baking soda
- ¼ teaspoon salt
- ½ cup solid extra-virgin coconut oil, plus more for pan
- ¼ cup unsweetened almond milk

FILLING

- 5 ripe peaches, peeled or unpeeled and pits removed, sliced ¼ inch thick
- 2 tablespoons maple syrup
- 1 tablespoon arrowroot

Preheat oven to 375°F.

Oil a 9-inch ovenproof skillet or 8 x 8-inch baking pan with coconut oil.

CRUST In a bowl, combine the flour, sugar, baking powder, baking soda, and salt. Fold in oil and milk. Using your hand, mix the ingredients until just incorporated (don't over mix it) and a thick dough is formed. The consistency will resemble cookie dough. Be careful not to over mix the dough or it will bake into a dryer biscuit.

FILLING In a large bowl, gently combine peaches and maple syrup. In a separate bowl, whisk ⅓ cup water with the arrowroot. Combine the arrowroot mixture with the peaches. Spread the peaches in the skillet or baking pan. Using your fingers, pinch off spoon-sized pieces of the dough and place them on top of the peach filling. Do not spread the dough; just place the pieces around to cover the top. The dough will expand slightly while baking. Place the skillet or pan in the oven and bake until the crust is golden brown, 30 to 35 minutes. Let the cobbler cool for 10 to 15 minutes and serve warm. It's delicious served with Maple Pecan Ice Cream (page 219).

TIP Gluten-free coconut flour can be substituted for white whole wheat flour.

MAKES 4 SERVINGS

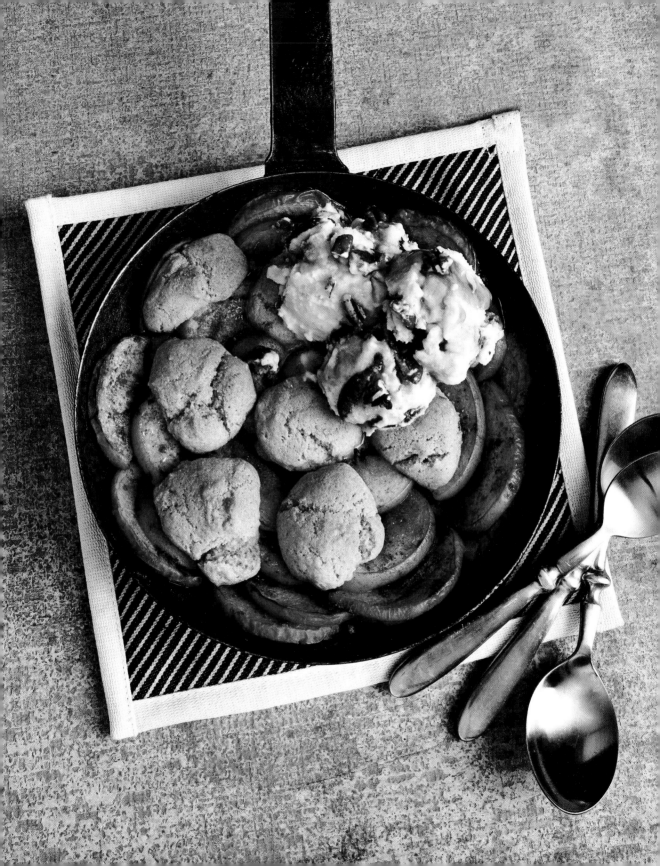

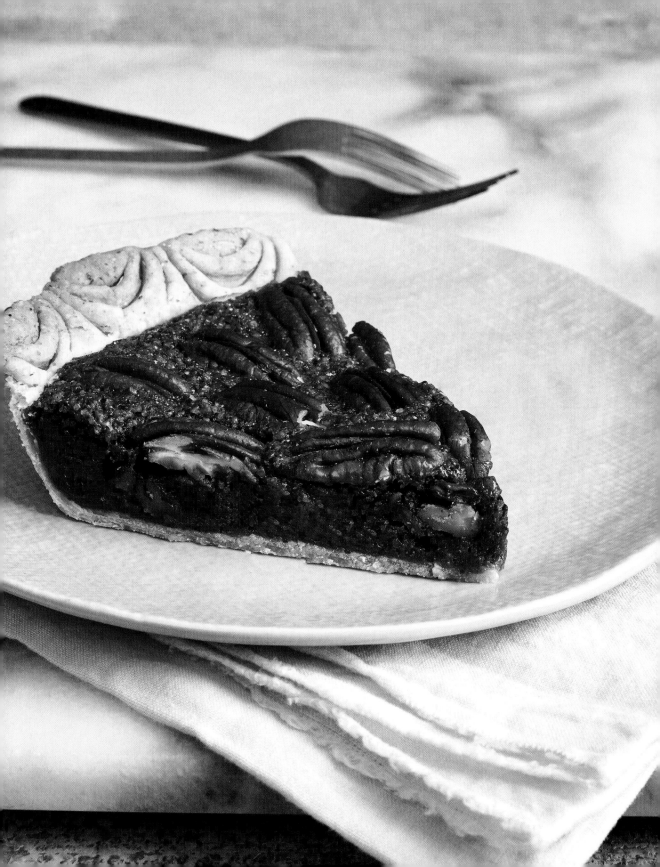

PERFECT PECAN PIE

My mom created this updated version of the pecan pie her mother used to make when she was growing up in South Carolina. It has everything you'd expect: a thick and gooey filling that's not too sweet, a caramelized topping with whole pecans pressed in, and a light and flaky crust. It's still delicious, just healthier. Pecans are the most antioxidant-rich tree nut—which includes antioxidant vitamins E and A that can help ward off free radicals that lead to premature aging of the skin.

Preheat oven to 350°F.

In a food processor, add 1 cup of the whole pecans and process until a coarse meal is formed. Place the meal in a medium bowl and add the chopped pecans. Stir until just combined. In a large bowl, combine the maple syrup, brown rice syrup, cinnamon, vanilla, flaxseed meal, milk, oil, and salt. Add the pecan mixture to the wet mixture and stir until mixed well. Stir in 1 tablespoon of the whole wheat flour at a time. You want the batter to be thick, but still loose enough to pour. Pour the batter into the pie crust. Arrange the remaining whole pecans on top. Bake for 45 minutes. Let the pie cool completely for the filling to firmly set. Serve immediately. Maple Pecan Ice Cream (page 219) or a dollop of Orange Cashew Cream (page 226) complement the pie beautifully.

TIP If you prefer a slightly less sweet pie, omit the brown rice syrup.

MAKES 7-9 SERVINGS

1¾ cups whole pecans
1 cup chopped pecans
¾ cup maple syrup
¼ cup brown rice syrup
½ teaspoon cinnamon
1 teaspoon vanilla
3 tablespoons ground flaxseed meal
¼ cup unsweetened almond milk
2 tablespoons extra-virgin coconut oil
⅛ teaspoon sea salt
2 tablespoons whole wheat flour
1 (9-inch) whole-grain pie crust

Apple Crumb Pie

This raw apple crumb pie is so quick, easy, and delicious that you'll be whipping it up again and again, especially during the hotter months when you don't want to turn on the oven. We all know that apples are good for us, and it's for good reason. Apples are among the most nutritious fruits, helping to reduce the risk for a wide range of chronic diseases, including heart disease, cancer, and diabetes, and promote overall health and longevity.

2 cups raw almonds
1 teaspoon sea salt
16 pitted Medjool dates, divided
1 large orange, peeled and seeds removed
5 firm medium apples, thinly chopped
2 tablespoons cinnamon

In a food processor, pulse the almonds, sea salt, and 10 of the dates until a crumbly mixture is formed and set aside.

In a blender, add the 6 remaining dates, the orange, and 2 teaspoons water and blend until smooth. If more water is needed to achieve a smooth consistency, add the water a half teaspoon at a time. Pour the syrup into a large bowl. Stir in the chopped apples and cinnamon. Spoon the filling into a 9-inch pie pan. Sprinkle the almond mixture on top of the apples and serve immediately. The pie tastes great with a dollop of Orange Cashew Cream (page 226) on top.

MAKES 8-10 SERVINGS

MAPLE PECAN ICE CREAM

This ice cream is truly divine. It has a delicious creaminess that will remind you of classic butter pecan ice cream—but without the butter. Coconut milk does the honors instead. This cholesterol-free ice cream also boasts skin-protecting vitamins A and E from the pecans. And just a note about equipment: you'll need a 13 x 9-inch stainless steel pan or an ice cream maker to freeze the ice cream.

PECANS Preheat oven to 250°F.

Line a baking sheet with parchment paper. In a small bowl, combine the pecans, maple syrup, and salt. Spread the pecans out on the baking sheet. Bake until the nuts start to turn darker brown, about 10 minutes, checking often to make sure they don't burn. When they're done, remove the pecans from the parchment paper and spread them onto wax paper to cool.

ICE CREAM In a blender, combine the milk and maple syrup. Blend for 30 seconds. In a separate bowl, combine the milk mixture and pecans. If using a 13 x 9-inch stainless steel pan, place the mixture in the pan. Cover with plastic wrap and place it in the freezer. Stir the ice cream thoroughly every 30 minutes until the ice cream is frozen. This will take about two to three hours. If using an ice cream maker, follow machine instructions. Serve frozen.

MAKES 4 SERVINGS

PECANS
- 1 cup raw pecan halves
- 1 tablespoon maple syrup
- ⅛ teaspoon sea salt

ICE CREAM
- 2 (13.5-ounce) cans coconut milk (light or regular)
- ¼ cup maple syrup

NO-BAKE CHOCOLATE PIE
with PISTACHIOS

In addition to being a chocolate lover's dream, this recipe makes a beautiful dessert. The light green pistachios look striking against the dark chocolate. And pistachios also give the pie a nutrient boost. Pistachios are the highest of all nuts in the antioxidants lutein and zeaxanthin, which promote eye health, and the second highest in protein (only almonds have more), and they help lower harmful LDL cholesterol levels, which promotes heart health. Avocados are another star ingredient here; they add richness as well as healthy fat.

CRUST

- 2 cups almond meal
- 8 Medjool dates, pitted and chopped (about ½ cup)
- Pinch sea salt

FILLING

- 4 ripe avocados, pitted
- 1 cup maple syrup
- 1 cup unsweetened cocoa powder
- ¼ cup extra-virgin coconut oil
- 1 teaspoon vanilla extract
- Pinch sea salt

GARNISH

- ¾ cup roughly chopped raw pistachios

CRUST Line the bottom of a 9-inch springform pan with parchment paper. Place almond meal, dates, 2 tablespoons water, and salt in a food processor. Process until mixture is finely ground and sticks together, about 30 seconds. Press almond mixture into the bottom of the lined pan and set aside.

FILLING Place avocado, maple syrup, cocoa powder, oil, vanilla, and salt in a blender. Blend until very smooth and creamy. Pour filling onto the pie crust and smooth with a spatula. Sprinkle the top with pistachios. Cover with plastic wrap and freeze for at least 3 hours. To thaw, place the pie in the refrigerator for at least 2 hours before serving. Because of the avocado, the pie is best served within several hours of removing it from the freezer. To remove from the pan, run a sharp knife around the edge. Serve cold or room temperature.

MAKES 8 SERVINGS

AGELESS ANTIOXIDANTS   BRAIN BOOSTER   HEALTH IS IN THE HUE   LONGEVITY LOVER
PROTEIN DREAM   SMOOTH SKIN   STRONG BONES   SUPER GREENS   VISION MISSION

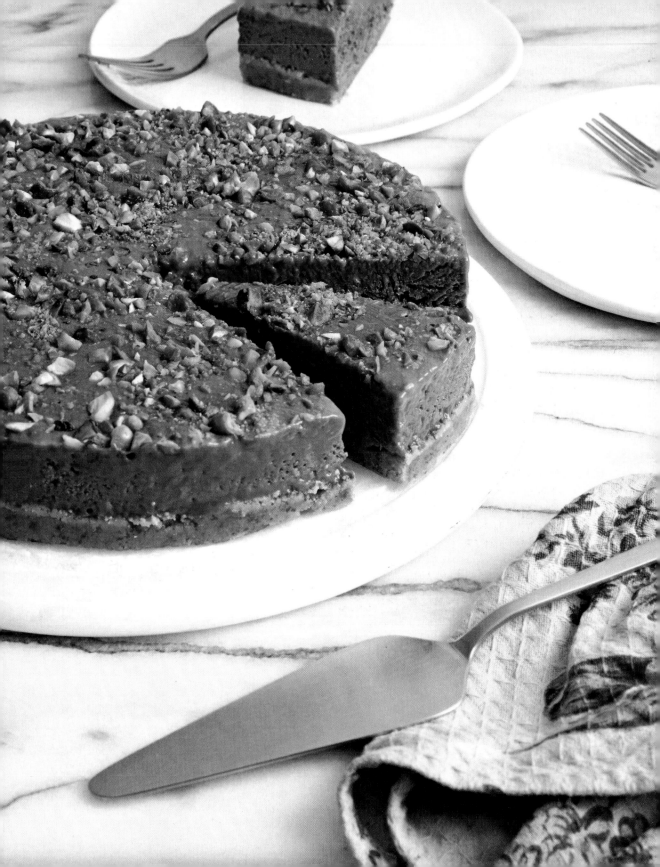

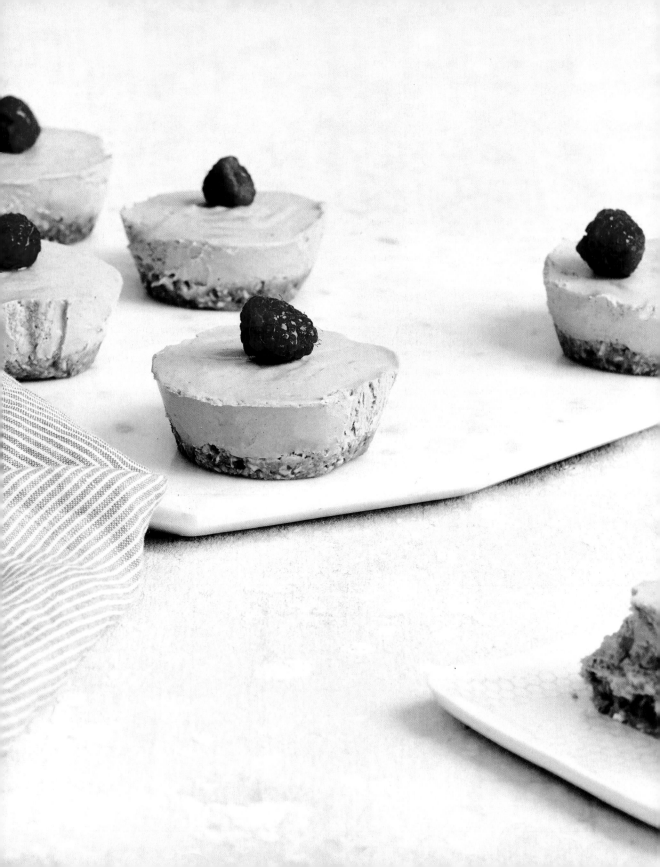

RASPBERRY
CHEESECAKE TARTLETS

These no-bake tartlets are the perfect size to indulge your taste for cheesecake in a healthier way. The combination of cashews and lemon juice is what provides the cheesecake's taste and texture. Cashews are a good source of copper, magnesium, and phosphorous, which help keep bones healthy.

CRUST Oil a 12-tin muffin pan (or use an unoiled 12-tin spring-form muffin pan) and set aside. In a food processor, combine the oats, dates, almond meal, 1½ tablespoons water, and salt. Process until mixture is evenly ground, sticky, and will hold together, about 1 minute. Divide the oat mixture evenly into the bottom of each tin. You can use the bottom of a glass that fits inside the muffin tin to press down the oatmeal mixture. If the mixture sticks to the glass, use a piece of parchment paper to cover the glass bottom and sides.

FILLING In a blender, combine the cashews, lemon juice, oil, syrup, raspberries, vanilla, salt, and 3 tablespoons water and blend until very smooth. If the mixture is too thick, add 1 teaspoon water at a time to make it thinner. Spoon the cashew mixture on top of the crust. Cover tightly with plastic wrap, and freeze for at least 3 hours. Let thaw slightly for 10 to 15 minutes in the refrigerator before serving. Leftover tartlets can be stored in heavy-duty freezer bags in the freezer for up to 2 weeks.

TIPS You can swap out lime juice for lemon juice with the same great cheesecake-taste results.

For a more classic cheesecake, you can add the raspberries as toppings and leave the filling fruit-free.

MAKES 8-12 TARTLETS

CRUST

- 1¼ cups rolled oats
- 12 Medjool dates, pitted and chopped (about ¾ cup)
- 3 tablespoons almond meal
  Pinch sea salt

FILLING

- 3 cups raw cashews, soaked in water for 1 hour and drained
- ½ cup freshly squeezed lemon juice (about 5 to 6 lemons)
- ¾ cup extra-virgin coconut oil
- ½ cup maple syrup
- 1 cup fresh raspberries
- 1 teaspoon vanilla extract
  Pinch sea salt

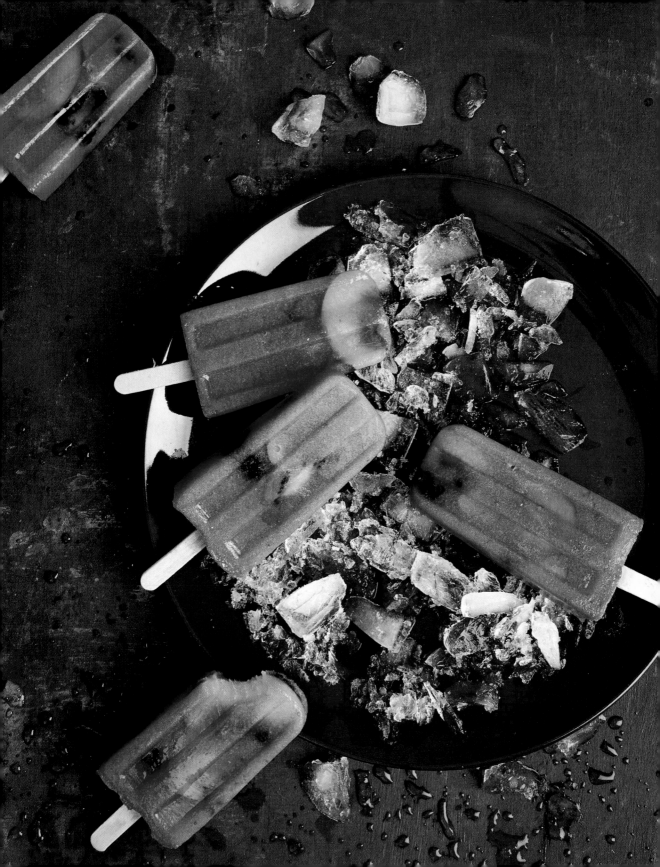

Fruity Ice Pops

These fruity ice pops are the ultimate summertime treat for kids and adults. The rainbow of antioxidant-rich fruits makes them a delicious example of Health Is in the Hue. Make them ahead of time so you'll have them on hand whenever the mood (or heat) strikes.

Place the kiwi, peaches, and blackberries equally (or unequally) in six ice pop molds. In a blender, combine the watermelon chunks and strawberries, and blend until smooth. Pour the purée into the molds. Freeze until solid, about 4 hours or more. Remove from the molds and serve immediately.

MAKES 6 ICE POPS

1 kiwi, peeled and cut into thin slices

1 peach, peeled and diced

½ cup blackberries

¼ medium watermelon, seedless or seeds removed, cut into chunks (about 3 cups)

½ pound fresh strawberries, hulls removed

PINEAPPLE CARROT CUPCAKES
with ORANGE CASHEW CREAM TOPPING

My mother and I are carrot cake connoisseurs. So when we created this recipe, we knew it had to be fabulous. These cupcakes are super moist, light and fluffy, and incredibly delicious. Loaded with carrots and pineapples and topped with a creamy cashew frosting, they're a healthier dessert you can feel good about.

ORANGE CASHEW CREAM

- 1 cup raw cashews, soaked overnight and drained
- 3 tablespoons maple syrup
- 2 tablespoons freshly squeezed orange juice (about ½ medium orange)
- 1 tablespoon extra-virgin coconut oil
- ½ teaspoon vanilla extract

CUPCAKES

- 1⅓ cups whole wheat pastry flour
- 1 cup whole wheat flour
- 2 tablespoons ground flaxseed meal
- 2 teaspoons baking powder
- 1 teaspoon baking soda
- 1 teaspoon arrowroot
- 2 teaspoons cinnamon
- 1 teaspoon nutmeg
- 1 teaspoon allspice
- ½ teaspoon ground cloves
- ⅓ cup extra-virgin coconut oil

- 1 cup maple syrup
- Pineapple juice reserved from canned pineapple (see below)
- 1 teaspoon vanilla extract
- 3 large carrots, finely grated (about 2 cups loosely packed)
- 1 (15-ounce) can of unsweetened crushed pineapple, with juice drained and reserved (should yield ⅓ to ½ cup)
- 1 cup chopped walnuts
- 1 cup raisins (optional)

RECIPE CONTINUED ON PAGE 228

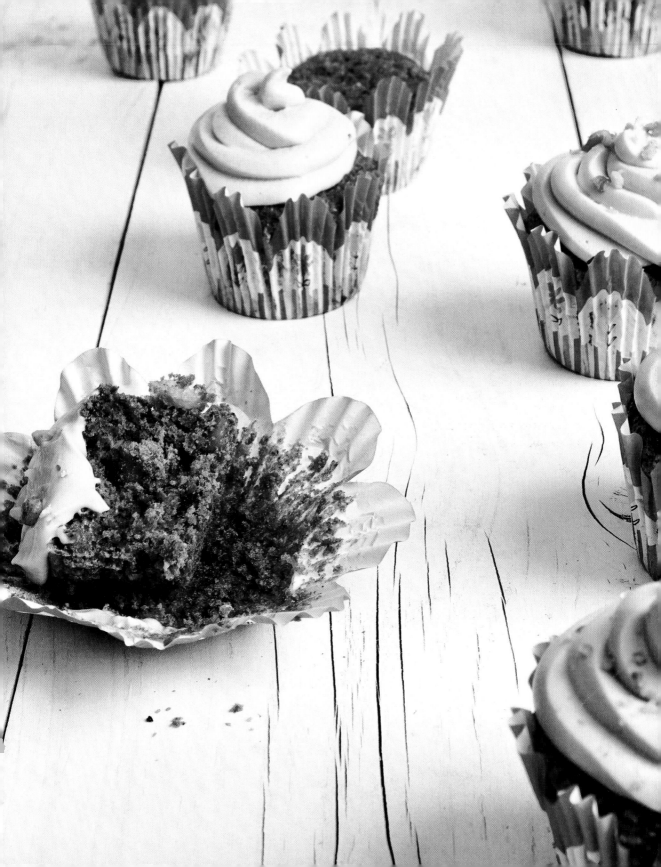

RECIPE CONTINUED FROM PAGE 226

Preheat oven to 350°F.

Line a cupcake tin with paper cups or oil the cupcake tin and set aside.

ORANGE CASHEW CREAM In a blender, combine all the ingredients and blend until smooth. (If needed, add 1 teaspoon of orange juice or water at a time to help with blending.) Place frosting in a bowl, cover, and chill in the freezer for 30 minutes to 1 hour to thicken.

CUPCAKES In a large bowl, sift together the whole wheat pastry flour and whole wheat flour. Add flaxseed meal, baking powder, baking soda, arrowroot, cinnamon, nutmeg, allspice, and cloves and whisk until thoroughly combined.

In a separate bowl, combine the oil, maple syrup, pineapple juice, and vanilla and mix thoroughly. Fold in the carrots and pineapple.

Gently fold the wet mixture into the dry mixture until just combined. Be sure not to over mix because that will lead to dry muffins. A few lumps here and there are fine. Fold in the walnuts and optional raisins. Spoon the batter into the muffin pan. Bake for 20 to 30 minutes, or until a toothpick inserted in the middle comes out clean. Let the cupcakes cool completely. Top the cupcakes with the cashew cream and serve.

MAKES 12 LARGE CUPCAKES

Almost Ambrosia

This recipe is a light and refreshing take on traditional ambrosia, without the heavy cream or marshmallows. In other words, it's a beautiful fruit salad topped with coconut flakes and nuts that you eat for dessert. And after all is said and done, sometimes a taste of fruit is the perfect ending to a really good meal.

1   banana, cut into ⅛-inch-thick slices

2   kiwis, peeled and cut into ⅛-inch-thick slices

Sections from 2 peeled blood oranges

1   cup red grapes, halved

½   medium pomegranate, seeds only (about ½ cup)

½   cup dried, unsweetened coconut flakes

¼   cup chopped raw pecans, chopped

In a large bowl, combine the banana, kiwis, oranges, grapes, and pomegranate seeds. Transfer to a glass bowl with a top and chill in the refrigerator for 30 minutes. Top with coconut flakes and pecans. Serve immediately.

MAKES 4 SERVINGS

METRIC CONVERSIONS

The recipes in this book have not been tested with metric measurements, so some variations might occur. Remember that the weight of dry ingredients varies according to the volume or density factor: 1 cup of flour weighs far less than 1 cup of sugar, and 1 tablespoon doesn't necessarily hold 3 teaspoons.

GENERAL FORMULA FOR METRIC CONVERSION

Ounces to grams.........multiply ounces by 28.35
Grams to ounces.........multiply ounces by 0.035
Pounds to grams ....multiply pounds by 453.5
Pounds to kilograms ...multiply pounds by 0.45
Cups to liters ....multiply cups by 0.24
Fahrenheit to Celsius ..subtract 32 from Fahrenheit temperature, multiply by 5, divide by 9
Celsius to Fahrenheit ..multiply Celsius temperature by 9, divide by 5, add 32

VOLUME (LIQUID) MEASUREMENTS

1 teaspoon = $\frac{1}{6}$ fluid ounce = 5 milliliters
1 tablespoon = $\frac{1}{2}$ fluid ounce = 15 milliliters
2 tablespoons = 1 fluid ounce = 30 milliliters
$\frac{1}{4}$ cup = 2 fluid ounces = 60 milliliters
$\frac{1}{3}$ cup = 2 $\frac{2}{3}$ fluid ounces = 79 milliliters
$\frac{1}{2}$ cup = 4 fluid ounces = 118 milliliters
1 cup or $\frac{1}{2}$ pint = 8 fluid ounces = 250 milliliters
2 cups or 1 pint = 16 fluid ounces = 500 milliliters
4 cups or 1 quart = 32 fluid ounces = 1,000 milliliters
1 gallon = 4 liters

VOLUME (DRY) MEASUREMENTS

$\frac{1}{4}$ teaspoon = 1 milliliter
$\frac{1}{2}$ teaspoon = 2 milliliters
$\frac{3}{4}$ teaspoon = 4 milliliters
1 teaspoon = 5 milliliters
1 tablespoon = 15 milliliters
$\frac{1}{4}$ cup = 59 milliliters
$\frac{1}{3}$ cup = 79 milliliters
$\frac{1}{2}$ cup = 118 milliliters
$\frac{2}{3}$ cup = 158 milliliters
$\frac{3}{4}$ cup = 177 milliliters
1 cup = 225 milliliters
4 cups or 1 quart = 1 liter
$\frac{1}{2}$ gallon = 2 liters
1 gallon = 4 liters

WEIGHT (MASS) MEASUREMENTS

1 ounce = 30 grams
2 ounces = 55 grams
3 ounces = 85 grams
4 ounces = $\frac{1}{4}$ pound = 125 grams
8 ounces = $\frac{1}{2}$ pound = 240 grams
12 ounces = $\frac{3}{4}$ pound = 375 grams
16 ounces = 1 pound = 454 grams

LINEAR MEASUREMENTS

$\frac{1}{2}$ in = 1 $\frac{1}{2}$ cm
1 inch = 2 $\frac{1}{2}$ cm
6 inches = 15 cm
8 inches = 20 cm
10 inches = 25 cm
12 inches = 30 cm
20 inches = 50 cm

OVEN TEMPERATURE EQUIVALENTS, FAHRENHEIT (F) AND CELSIUS (C)

100°F = 38°C
200°F = 95°C
250°F = 120°C
300°F = 150°C
350°F = 180°C
400°F = 205°C
450°F = 230°C

RESOURCES

Adams, Carol J., et al. 2014. *Never Too Late to Go Vegan: The Over-50 Guide to Adopting and Thriving on a Plant-Based Diet.* New York: The Experiment.

Appleby, P. N., et al. 2011. "Diet, Vegetarianism, and Cataract Risk." *American Journal of Clinical Nutrition* 93 (5): 1128–1135.

Ford, E. S., et al. 2009. "Healthy Living Is the Best Revenge: Findings from the European Prospective Investigation into Cancer and Nutrition–Potsdam Study." *Archives of Internal Medicine* 169 (15):1355–1362.

Greger, Michael. 2015. *How Not to Die: Discover the Foods Scientifically Proven to Prevent and Reverse Disease.* New York: Flatiron Books.

McQuirter, Tracye. 2010. *By Any Greens Necessary: A Revolutionary Guide for Black Women Who Want to Eat Great, Get Healthy, Lose Weight, and Look Phat.* Chicago: Chicago Review Press.

Murray, C. J., et al. 2013. "The State of US Health, 1999–2010: Burden of Diseases, Injuries, and Risk Factors." *Journal of the American Medical Association* 310 (6): 591–608.

Nagata, C., et al. 2010. "Association of Dietary Fat, Vegetables and Antioxidant Micronutrients with Skin Ageing in Japanese Women." *British Journal of Nutrition* 103 (10):1493–1498.

Rizzo, N. S., et al. 2013. "Nutrient Profiles of Vegetarian and Nonvegetarian Dietary Patterns." *Journal of the Academy of Nutrition and Dietetics* 113 (12):1610–1619.

"Survey of Vegans 2013: The Results." http://thevegantruth.blogspot.com/2013/09/survey-of-vegans-2013-results_13html.

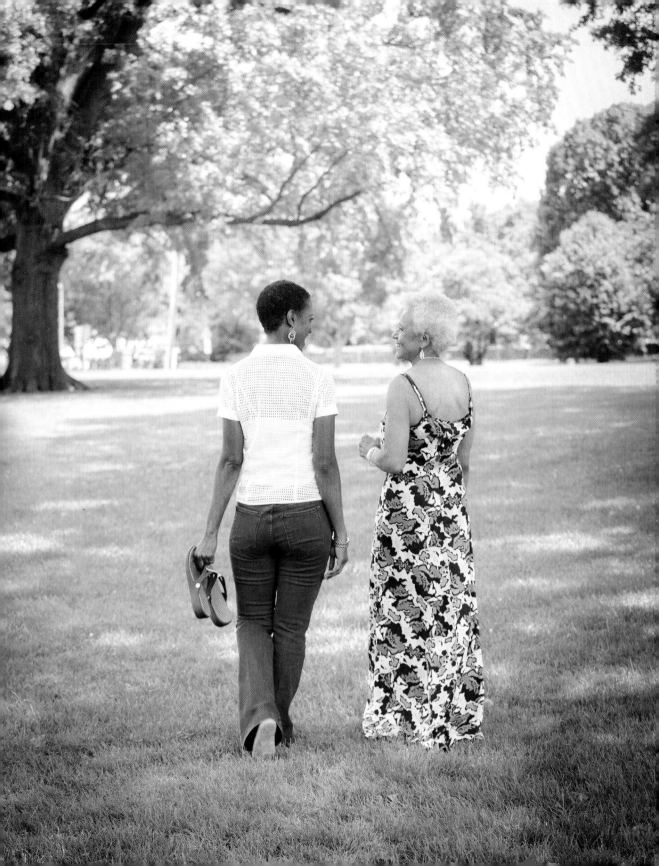

ACKNOWLEDGMENTS

To my mother, Mary McQuirter, thank you for working with me on this book. Creating and testing recipes with you in the kitchen while we listened to Motown was a beautiful experience that I'll always treasure. And I know that your vegan journey will be an inspiration to everyone who reads this book for years to come.

To my sister, Marya McQuirter, and my niece, Mara, thank you for tasting so many of these recipes and providing invaluable feedback, and for your encouragement throughout the process. Thank you to my sister, Veronica Hale, for always being so supportive, for your good advice, and helping me stay on track. And to my nieces, Raneesha and Taylor, thank you for your encouraging words. And to my extended family, a special shout out for all of your continued love and support. Thanks for always lifting me up.

To my agent, Lindsay Edgecombe, thank you for your excitement about this book from the beginning and your extraordinary guidance and support throughout the journey to completion. To my editor, Renee Sedliar, thank you for your unwavering commitment and passion for this project, and for all of your brilliant editing. And thanks to the entire team at Hachette for your incredible work on the book and for making the publishing process so seamless.

Thank you to Kate Lewis for your gorgeous food photography and styling. I'm grateful for your amazing work and enthusiasm for this book. To Delores Holloway, thank you for your stunning cover photography and for capturing the beautiful lifestyle shots of me and my mother. Thank you to Robin Fisher for your gifted personal styling and vision for the photo shoots.

To my dream team of recipe testers, I'm grateful for your dedication, time, and constructive feedback. It made all the difference. Thank you to Nadia Stevens for going above and beyond with your impeccable catering as well as recipe tasting. And my deepest gratitude to Cassandra Barber, Beverly Hilbert, Annette Harris Powell, Carolyn Woods, Valeria Villasenor-Bruyere, Monique Koch, Monique Flowers, LaCara Reddick, and Saundra Woods. And thank you to Sidra Forman for helping to develop recipes for the book.

To my friends Kristine Louis, Leslie Riley, Gina Lilavois, Carmen Scott, Kurtis Patterson, Barbara Agyeman, Susan Vitka, and those of you whom I already mentioned above as recipe testers, thank you for cheerleading, listening, and helping me stay the course during my book-writing journey. I truly appreciate you.

And finally, thank you to all the wonderful people I've met through my work over the last thirty years. Each time you greet me with a big smile or a warm hug and say that my work has helped change your life, I feel honored and just plain happy! You inspire me to keep on sharing, learning, and growing.

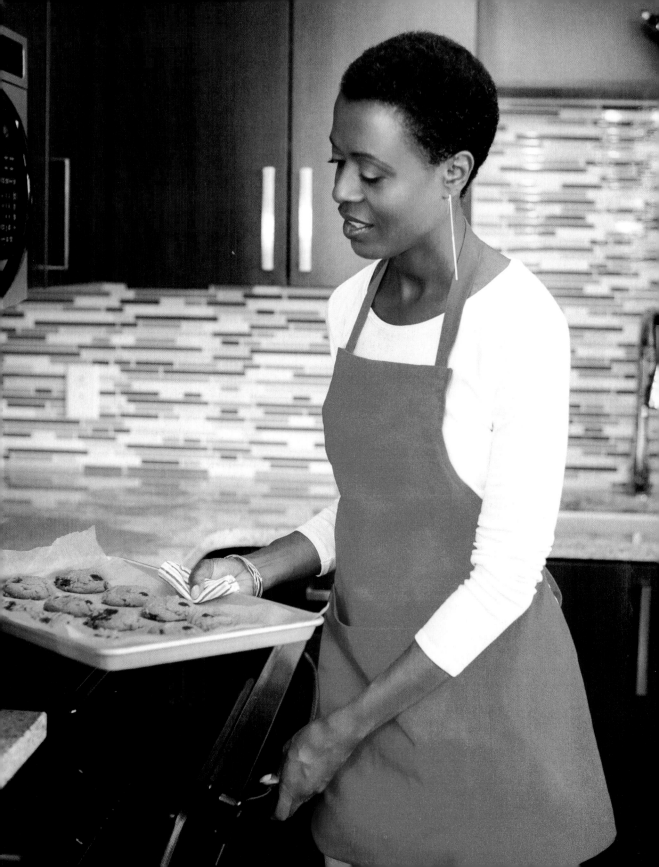

INDEX

italics indicate photographs.

ABOUT THE AUTHORS

TRACYE MCQUIRTER, MPH, was named a national food hero changing the way America eats for the better by *Vegetarian Times* and her best-selling book, *By Any Greens Necessary*, established her as one of the most influential vegans in the country. As a writer, speaker, public health nutritionist, and thirty-year vegan, Tracye has been teaching people how and why to live a healthy vegan lifestyle for the past twenty-five years. She recently created the first-of-its-kind, free African American Vegan Starter Guide in partnership with Farm Sanctuary. Previously, she co-created one of the earliest vegan websites twenty years ago, which was also the first by and for African American vegans. Tracye directed the nation's first federally funded vegan nutrition program and was a nutrition advisor for the Black Women's Health Imperative. As an adjunct professor at the University of the District of Columbia, Tracye designed and taught a plant-based nutrition curriculum for the District of Columbia Public Schools System to help prevent and reverse childhood obesity in Washington, DC. She is a cofounder of We Feed People and the Community Support Network, and advisory board member of Coalition for Healthy School Food, Black Vegans Rock, PlantPure Nation Foundation, and Hip Hop is Green. Her work has been featured in *The New York Times*, *The Washington Post*, *Essence*, *Bon Appetit*, *Ebony*, *VegNews*, *The Huffington Post*, *Black Enterprise, and more*. She is a graduate of Sidwell Friends School, Amherst College, and New York University, where she received a master's degree in public health nutrition. You can find Tracye on social media at ByAnyGreensNecessary.com and @byanygreens.

MARY DAVIS MCQUIRTER is a thirty-year vegan who continues to be healthy, fit, and active into her eighties. She has been retired from Covington and Burling law firm for twenty years and has been an active volunteer for more than forty years, helping children, abused women, mentally ill adults, and families in need. Mary also co-founded the Community Support Network, a nonprofit organization that developed programs to serve the needs of her community for more than twenty years. Mary has also worked with her daughter, Tracye, to teach vegan nutrition classes for seniors in Washington, DC. As an avid quilter, Mary currently teaches quilting classes at her local senior wellness center, where she also takes exercise classes five days a week (at least twice a day).

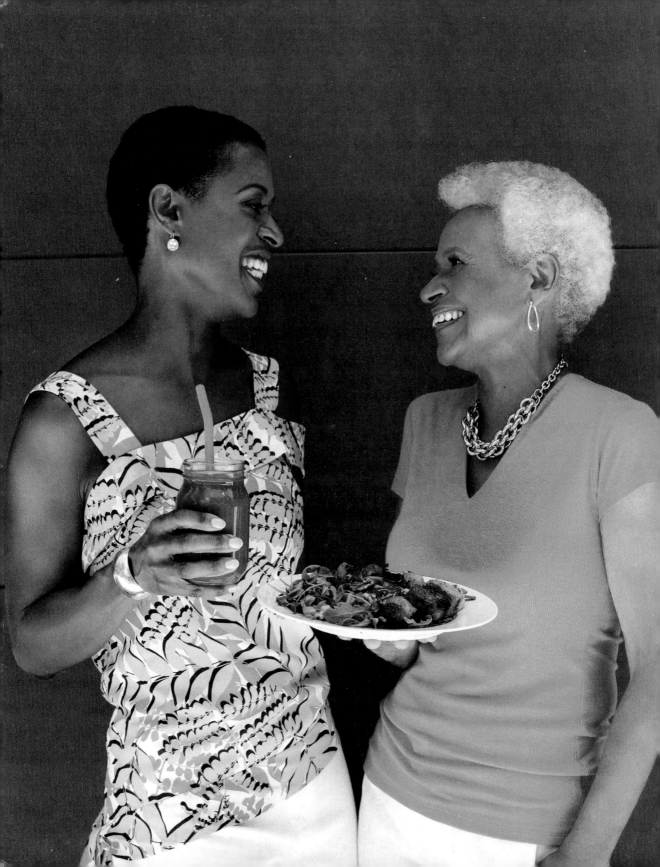